The Low Iodine Diet
COOKBOOK

Easy and Delicious Recipes and
Tips for Thyroid Cancer Patients

Norene Gilletz author of *Healthy Helpings*

Introduction by Kenneth Ain, M.D., Director,
Thyroid Oncology Program, University of Kentucky

YOUR HEALTH PRESS | Amazon Edition

The Low Iodine Diet Cookbook: Easy and Delicious Recipes and Tips for Thyroid Cancer Patients
Your Health Press

Important Notice:
The purpose of this book is to educate. It is sold with the understanding that the author and publisher shall have neither liability nor responsibility for any injury caused or alleged to be caused directly or indirectly by the information contained in this book. While every effort has been made to ensure its accuracy, the book's contents should not be construed as medical advice. Each person's health needs are unique. To obtain recommendations appropriate to your particular situation, please consult a qualified healthcare provider. The low iodine diet is not a diet for the general public, but a specific, temporary diet for thyroid cancer patients.

Design of print and digital editions: Anita Janik-Jones
Cover recipe: Grilled London Broil (recipe page 170)
Cover photo: istockphoto.com

ISBN 978-0-9851568-4-8

OTHER BOOKS BY NORENE GILLETZ

The New Food Processor Bible: 30th Anniversary Edition, Whitecap (2011)

The Frequent Fiber Cookbook: Delicious Recipes and Tips for People on a High Fiber Diet, Your Health Press (2007)

Norene's Healthy Kitchen, Whitecap (2007)

Healthy Helpings, Whitecap (2006)

The PCOS Diet Cookbook: Delicious Recipes and Tips for Women with PCOS on the Low GI Diet, Your Health Press (2007)

Second Helpings, Please!, Gourmania (1968)

TABLE OF CONTENTS

Table of Contents

WHAT IS THE LOW IODINE DIET AND WHY DO YOU NEED IT?

Kenneth B. Ain, M.D.

Professor of Medicine, Director, Thyroid Oncology Program, Division of Endocrinology and Molecular Medicine, University of Kentucky Medical Center, and Director, Thyroid Cancer Research Laboratory, Veterans Affairs Medical Center, Lexington, KY.

Thyroid cancer is an unusual type of cancer. Thyroid cancer and most other cancers are treated with surgery to remove as much of the tumor as possible. However, there are frequently tiny bits of tumor, too small to be seen by the surgeon or found with x-ray pictures or scans, which the surgeon is unable to find or remove. Sometimes tumor cells have spread to other parts of the body beyond the neck region. In some other cancers, the tiny residual bits of tumor are treated with chemotherapy, drugs that are intended to poison these tumor bits without hurting normal parts of the body. Thyroid cancer, on the other hand, cannot currently be treated with chemotherapy to kill the tumor cells.

Instead, more than half a century ago, clever physicians figured out a different way to find residual thyroid cancer (tumor bits). Realizing that normal thyroid cells have a phenomenal ability to suck up iodine (thyroid cells "suck up" iodine in order to make thyroid hormone), they reasoned that thyroid *cancer* cells would also be able to suck up iodine. Their idea was to give thyroid cancer patients small doses of radioactive iodine after their surgery, which would permit these physicians to "see" where bits of thyroid cancer remained or had spread to in their patients' bodies. They used scanning machines to view the radioactive "glow" from these thyroid cancer bits containing radioactive iodine. Even more important, they found that larger doses of radioactive iodine would kill these bits of thyroid cancer, anywhere they might have spread, without harming most normal body parts.

How does iodine get into thyroid cancer cells?

How do normal thyroid cells and thyroid cancer cells suck up iodine? These tiny cells make small iodine "pumps," called sodium-iodide symporters, which are placed in the cell membrane ("skin") of these cells, immediately start sucking up iodine from the blood. A special hormone, *thyroid stimulating hormone*, or TSH, naturally produced by the pituitary gland, stimulates each of these cells to produce these iodine pumps. TSH is normally released by the pituitary gland in response to low thyroid hormone levels. This is why, after surgically removing your thyroid gland (known as a thyroidectomy), the traditional method of preparing you for a radioactive iodine scan or therapy requires you to withhold taking thyroid hormone medication. This is an effective way to sufficiently increase the TSH level to cause thyroid cancer cells, wherever they may have travelled, to produce enough iodine pumps to be able to suck up radioactive iodine. However, the hypothyroid condition that ensues can sometimes be very debilitating.

An alternative to stopping thyroid hormone medication, while still having sufficiently high levels of TSH to permit thyroid cancer cells to suck up radioactive iodine effectively, is to take TSH as a medication. This TSH is given as an injection (Thyrogen®) in two or three doses, and can be taken while continuing to take thyroid hormone medication, thereby avoiding any hypothyroid symptoms. Your physician should be aware of the appropriate situations for using Thyrogen® or using a hypothyroid preparation method.

Why do we need to decrease dietary iodine?

Raising your TSH level is only part of the preparation for effective use of radioactive iodine when dealing with thyroid cancer. It's important to "starve" the cancer cells of the relatively large quantities of non-radioactive iodine in your body. This allows the radioactive iodine to enter them. Your thyroid cancer cells can't tell the difference between iodine that is radioactive and iodine that is non-radioactive ("stable" iodine).

Stable iodine enters your body through your *diet*. Many parts of the developing world have problems with iodine deficiency, and as a result people in these regions suffer from hypothyroidism and associated medical problems. In most industrialized countries, great effort has been made to prevent these problems by supplementing iodine in the diet through *iodized salt*. Additional iodine enters our diet from fish, seafood, kelp, dairy products, artificial red food dye (FD&C Red Dye #3) and multivitamins. This dietary iodine is considered healthy for most people; however, it's *not* needed in people whose thyroid glands have been removed and who take thyroid hormone as a medication.

Typical amounts of dietary iodine can interfere with the use of radioactive iodine for thyroid cancer. The reason for this is as follows.

An "average" daily amount of dietary iodine in North America is approximately 500 micrograms (mcg). This number can be lower in vegetarians who don't consume any animal products (vegans), and much higher in lovers of sushi and seafood. It can exceed several thousand micrograms in people after an injection of intravenous contrast dye for a CT scan, and this can last for up to 10 months after a single injection. (You or your doctor can look up the following research article as a source for this information: Spate, V.L., Morris, J.S., Nichols, T.A., et al., 1998."Longitudinal study of iodine in toenails following IV administration of an iodine-containing contrast agent." *Journal of Radioanalytical and Nuclear Chemistry.* 236:71-76.)

This amount of stable iodine in your body may seem inconsequential until you learn that the amount of radioactive iodine in a treatment or scanning dose is usually only 2 mcg. These 2 mcg of iodine are highly radioactive, but don't actually constitute much iodine. Taken within the context of the typical total body pool of iodine in one day, 2 mcg (radioactive iodine) of 502 mcg (total iodine) means that only 0.4 percent of the iodine in your body is radioactive.It follows that if a thyroid cancer cell in your body sucks up 1,000 iodine atoms, only four of them are radioactive. Certainly this isn't a very effective way to find these cells with a scan, or treat them with the radioactive iodine.

On the other hand, if you follow a **Low Iodine Diet** (or **LID**, as described in this book) prior to receiving your 2 mcg dose of radioactive iodine, your daily total iodine intake decreases—from 500 mcg to less than 40 mcg. In this case, the radioactive iodine constitutes 2 mcg of 42 mcg of iodine, meaning that at least five percent of the iodine in your body is radioactive. The same thyroid cancer cell as in the paragraph above, sucking up 1000 iodine atoms, would then take in at least 50 radioactive iodine atoms. This results in more than 12 times the amount of radioactivity in each thyroid cancer cell, using a **LID**, with everything else being the same (same treatment or scan dose, same hypothyroid or Thyrogen® preparation), as compared to following your usual diet.

The ability of a **LID** to enhance radioactive iodine uptake in thyroid cancer cells is more than merely speculative. In my two decades as a thyroid oncologist, I've seen many patients who were sent to me because they were labeled as being "radioactive iodine unresponsive" or having "negative" radioactive iodine scans *despite having known residual thyroid cancer*. With many of them, careful evaluations of their medical histories revealed that *they were not prepared with a LID or had recently been given an iodine contrast dye for a CT scan*. When suitably prepared with a **LID**, in many cases, their tumors were able to suck up (concentrate) radioactive iodine well enough to reliably scan and sometimes treat them. More often, following a **LID** for the first time significantly enhanced previous marginal amounts of radioactive iodine uptake into tumors.

In assessing the ability of a **LID** to increase radioactive iodine uptake, it's necessary to know that the diet is sufficiently low in iodine to truly be a **LID**. In rare studies claiming to evaluate a **LID** (for example, see: Morris, L.F., Wilder, M.S., Waxman, A.D., Braunstein, G.D., 2001. "Re-evaluation of the impact of a stringent low iodine diet on ablation rates in radioiodine treatment of thyroid carcinoma." *Thyroid*. 11:749-55), the actual diet was not sufficiently low in iodine to give a valid appraisal of its effect. In studies that use a good **LID** (such as: Pluijmen, M.J., Eustatia-Rutten, C., Goslings, B.M., et al., 2003. "Effects of low-iodide diet on postsurgical radioiodide ablation therapy in patients with differentiated thyroid carcinoma." *Clinical Endocrinology (Oxford)*. 58:428-35), the enhancements of radioactive iodine concentration into tumor cells are clearly demonstrated.

Note: *Throughout this book, we use the term "iodine," even when the proper term is "iodide," to avoid confusion. Iodine is the name of the element, while iodide is the ionic form of iodine usually present in body fluids.*

HISTORY OF THE LOW IODINE DIET

In the more than half-century physicians have used radioactive iodine to treat thyroid cancer, they have long appreciated the need to enhance the effectiveness of this treatment. As early as 1969, diuretics were used in an attempt to deplete patients of dietary iodine (see: Hamburger, J.I., 1969. "Diuretic augmentation of 131I uptake in inoperable thyroid cancer." *New England Journal of Medicine*. 280:1091-94); however, current practices find them to be less useful than a good **LID**. Thyroid cancer specialists were aware of the value of a **LID** for many years (you or your doctor can look up: Maxon, H.R., Thomas, S.R., Boehringer, A., et al., 1983. "Low iodine diet in I-131 ablation of thyroid remnants." *Clinical Nuclear Medicine*. 8:123-26), although many of them couldn't agree on the composition of the diet. This became easier after a group at the National Institutes of Health (NIH) in Bethesda, MD, proposed a simple diet that proved to be effective (see: Lakshmanan, M., Schaffer, A., Robbins, J., Reynolds, J., Norton, J., 1988. "A simplified low iodine diet in I-131 scanning and therapy of thyroid cancer." *Clinical Nuclear Medicine*. 13:866-68). I first learned of this diet during my thyroid cancer practice at the NIH and have made only a few changes to it in the ensuing years.

This **LID** remained relatively unknown to most physicians and thyroid cancer patients throughout the 1990s. In early 1997, I was invited to be a medical advisor on the Thyroid Cancer Survivors' Association (ThyCa) e-mail listserv, started by Karen Ferguson with later help from Dr. Arturo R. Rolla, and I provided its members with the **LID**, as well as information on the virtues of its use. ThyCa was instrumental in spreading the word regarding the **LID** to its membership. Most of the physicians treating ThyCa members first learned of the diet from their patients. ThyCa expanded from a listserv to a full-fledged patient-led organization under the leadership of the late Ric Blake in late 1997, then had its first Thyroid Cancer Survivors' Conference in 1998. The **LID** was posted on the ThyCa website, followed by a patient-generated recipe exchange. This helped educate large numbers of thyroid cancer patients and their physicians.

The Low Iodine Diet Cookbook by **Norene Gilletz** takes the process a large step forward. A culinary expert and renowned cookbook author, Norene Gilletz has used her talents to provide patients with a healthy and good-tasting approach to this diet. It's an approach that will enhance quality of life and medical care during a stressful time in the life of any thyroid cancer patient.

THE BASIC LOW IODINE DIET

The basic **LID** is summarized on the following instruction sheet that is provided to each of my own patients and circulated widely to many physicians and patient groups. It consists primarily of a list of restricted dietary items that contain relatively high amounts of stable iodine. The assumption is that anything that isn't restricted should be considered safe to eat as part of a balanced and varied diet. Unfortunately, these instructions make figuring out interesting foods that are appropriate to eat a matter of individual creativity. *This cookbook provides a solution to that problem.*

LOW IODINE DIET DIRECTIONS
Used for Preparation for Radioiodine Scans or Therapy

Avoid the following foods, starting when instructed prior to your radioactive iodine test, and continuing until a full day after your radioactive iodine treatment is completed.

1. Iodized salt, sea salt (*non-iodized* salt may be used).
2. Dairy products (milk, cheese, cream, yogurt, ice cream, butter).
3. Eggs (specifically avoid egg yolks; *egg whites* may be used).
4. Seafood (both fresh and salt-water fish, shellfish, seaweed, kelp).
5. Foods that contain the additives carrageen, agar-agar, algin, alginates.
6. Cured and corned foods (e.g., ham, corned beef, sausage, luncheon meats, sauerkraut, pickles).
7. Bread products that contain iodate dough conditioners (sometimes small bakery breads are safe; better to bake it yourself from scratch).
8. Foods and medications that contain *red* food dyes (specifically, FD&C Red Dye # 3; consult your physician about discontinuing or substituting for any red colored medicines).
9. Chocolate (because of the milk content). Non-dairy chocolate, however, is fine (see page 244 for more information).
10. Molasses.
11. Soy products (soy sauce, soy milk, tofu, edamame, soybeans). Soy lecithin and soybean oil is permitted.
12. Multivitamins (iodine content varies widely)

Additional Guidelines
1. Avoid restaurant foods, since there's no reliable way to determine what's in the food you order (see chapter 3 for dining out tips).
2. Use only LID-safe breads (e.g. breads you baked yourself with non-iodized salt) or bread substitutes, such as unsalted Matzo or unsalted tortillas (See Chapter 1).
3. Use non-iodized salt as desired (see "Getting Creative with Non-iodized Salts" on page 242).
4. *Always* read ingredients lists of prepared or packaged foods carefully.
5. Use olive oil as a condiment or in cooking in place of butter.

6. Prepare low iodine meals in advance if you wish, and freeze them for easy later use.

Important Note:

Food prepared from any fresh or frozen *meats, poultry, vegetables, and fruits* should be fine for this diet, provided that you don't add any of the ingredients listed, which you must avoid. Be careful of meat or poultry that's been injected with broth or preservative liquids. The diet is easiest when food is prepared from *basic ingredients*.

Strict adherence to this diet will significantly enhance the sensitivity of the radioiodine scans and the effectiveness of any radioiodine treatments.

AVOIDING UNNECESSARY RESTRICTIONS

This diet does *not* restrict *sodium* or salt. It only restricts *iodized* salt or sea salt (very likely to have iodine). Any salt that is labeled as not being iodized may be used freely. With respect to Kosher salts, some are non-iodized, while some contain iodine, so be sure to check labels. The problem with prepared foods that contain salt as an ingredient is that food labels do not state whether this salt is iodized or not. Manufacturers may not know whether they use iodized salt or non-iodized salt, and this may change without notification. For this reason, it's safer to avoid any foods that have salt listed as an ingredient. Instead, add your own non-iodized salt as desired. Many foods that contain significant amounts of sodium do not contain added salt or iodine. As long as salt is not listed as an ingredient, there is no reason to worry about the effects of iodized salt.

Erythrosine, listed as FD&C Red Dye #3, contains large quantities of stable iodine (see: Vought, R.L., Brown, F.A., Wolff, J., 1972. "Erythrosine: an adventitious source of iodide." *Journal of Clinical Endocrinology and Metabolism.* 34:747-52). Any food item with artificial red food coloring may contain Red Dye #3, unless specifically listed as containing some other red food dye. Sometimes purple colored items contain blue and red dyes; likewise, orange items have yellow and red dyes. Any time the artificial coloring is not specified, assume that it may contain Red Dye #3; but if the ingredients list is specific and lists other dyes, there is no reason to avoid the item unless other iodine-containing ingredients are present. Medication problems may also arise, as is the case with calcitriol (Rocaltrol®) in the 0.5 mcg size capsule, which contains Red Dye #3. This medication is commonly used to treat low calcium levels after thyroid surgery. Fortunately, the 0.25 mcg size capsule is free of Red Dye #3, and two of these substitute nicely for the larger capsule.

Some patients and physicians, although well intentioned, have mistakenly taken this diet to *unnecessary extremes*. They claim that specific types of beans, rice, vegetables or fruit (e.g., rhubarb) should be avoided. Sometimes they grow unduly concerned about tap water and potato skins. One problem is that many of the tables and assays for the iodine content of foods, beyond the stipulations of the basic **LID**, are unreliable due to the difficulties in testing for iodine. Another problem is that a good **LID** is *not* a *no* iodine diet. As long as the basic **LID** is followed (as aided by this cookbook), the amount of iodine ingested in a 24-hour period should be under 50 mcg. One way to assess this is to collect all of the urine you produce in a 24-hour period. The total amount of iodine in that urine sample reflects the total amount eaten during that time. In a variety of clinical trials, I've measured urine samples in many patients following the basic **LID** and found it to be highly reliable without unnecessary additional restrictions. In this cookbook you'll find recipes with all types of beans, potato skins, rice and rhubarb, which you should enjoy and not worry about.

Another area of confusion is soy lecithin. There are several reasons for this. First, most commercial lecithin is associated with soy sources, which suggests that there might be some iodine present, or that it might block cells from taking in iodine (goitrogenic). However, soy lecithin is extracted from soy oil, rather than the protein parts, and has just trace amounts of soy proteins (only enough to bother people with soy allergies). Soy oil, in reasonable amounts (usually as part of a vegetable oil mixture or a minor ingredient) won't add any discernible iodine to the diet and is not goitrogenic (blocking iodine uptake). There is no reason to think that soy lecithin is in any way unsafe for the **LID**. The major reason for misconceptions regarding lecithin and iodine has to do with the term "iodine number." This is an organic chemistry term meaning "a number expressing the percentage of iodine absorbed by a substance; performed as a measure of the proportion of unsaturated linkages present and usually determined in the analysis of oils and fats." The "iodine number" has *nothing* to do with *content* of iodine and is merely a laboratory test used when analyzing lecithin. So, don't worry if the label of your food item lists lecithin.

How long should I follow the Low Iodine Diet?

I typically advise my patients to start the **LID** two weeks before taking the radioactive iodine scan or treatment dose. For experienced people who are well versed in the **LID**, a week on the diet may be sufficient; however, most people make errors for the first week, requiring two weeks to reliably lower their stable iodine level. There is no advantage to spending longer periods of time on this diet prior to receiving radioactive iodine. Likewise, making significant errors while on the diet, just *one* day before receiving a radioactive iodine dose, will undo all of the good intentions of the entire two weeks on the **LID**.

When should you stop the LID and resume your usual diet?

There is no need to follow a **LID** longer than 24 hours after swallowing a radioactive iodine treatment dose. This is because the entire effective uptake of radioactive iodine into thyroid cancer cells is finished by this time, making any further **LID** efforts unnecessary. There is no need to prolong the **LID** further, even if a scan (a "post-therapy" scan) is performed at a later date. It may be necessary, however, to prolong the **LID** for two or three days after taking the radioactive iodine scan dose until all of the diagnostic scans are completed and a decision is made regarding whether a radioactive iodine treatment dose is to be given. Nonetheless, once a decision has been made to not give a radioiodine treatment dose, or 24 hours after the treatment dose has been given, there is no need to continue the **LID**.

Why can't I drink milk? Can I drink goat milk instead?

The iodine content in milk varies several-fold from place-to-place, month-to-month, and year-to-year. Animal feeding practices, veterinary medications and food processing techniques also affect it. For example, a study of commercial milk samples in 1978 in the U.S. showed variations from 360 mcg/liter to 1,320 mcg/liter (you or your doctor can look up: Park, Y.K., Harland, B.F., Vanderveen, J.E., Shank F.R., Prosky, L., 1981. "Estimation of dietary iodine intake of Americans in recent years." *Journal of the American Dietetics Association*. 79:17-24). The trends in iodine content in milk have shown increases over time, so *it's likely that current iodine values for milk are much higher*. For this reason, it's possible that a single teaspoon of milk may contain more than a quarter of the total daily iodine level aimed for in the low iodine diet. Considering that dietary compliance is rarely 100 percent for all other constituents (and that even "low iodine" food items contain some iodine), I suggest that it's prudent to avoid all dairy products during the diet. (Several milk substitutes and baking substitutes can be found in this cookbook.) Thus, I've given the following advice to my patients and to thyroid cancer patients on my listserv:

Do *not* use *any* milk from *any* mammal in *any* form. It doesn't matter if it's cow, goat, dog, whale, human, cat, pig, giraffe, monkey, hippopotamus, prairie dog, dolphin, or muskrat milk. It doesn't matter if it's fresh, fermented, powdered, frozen, shaken, stirred, dried, diluted, or coagulated. It doesn't matter if it's yogurt, cheese, ice cream, skim, whole, cream, or butter.

The glandular breast tissue of female mammals is able to transport and concentrate iodine from the bloodstream of the animal and produce milk with a relatively high iodine content. One can see how important this source of iodine might be for infant animals who depend on this iodine source for their own production of thyroid hormone. On top of all of this, commercial dairies use iodine-containing liquids to clean the teats of dairy animals. Similar liquids are used to clean the myriad tubing of milking equipment. All of these natural and unnatural processes add to the high iodine content of all *milk* and *milk products*.

How about vitamins?

Since iodine is a critical component of a healthy diet in people with thyroid glands, it's not surprising that most multivitamins provide iodine, usually as much as 150 mcg per tablet. Although exhaustive research might yield a few multivitamins that don't have iodine, it's not necessary to worry about missing vitamins for the one to three weeks, at most, that you will be on the **LID**.

What about injected CT scan dye? How do I tell when it's passed out of my body?

All CT (computerized axial tomography) scan contrast dyes, also used for angiograms and cardiac catheterizations, contain large amounts of stable iodine that will prevent thyroid cancer cells from sucking up radioactive iodine. Some of these contrast dyes are labeled as "*non-ionic*," confusing both physicians and patients into wrongly believing that they're free of iodine; however, *all of them contain large amounts of iodine*. Stable iodine contamination from this contrast dye is certainly an important actual and potential contribution to radioactive iodine scan and treatment failures. If you're given this contrast dye during the course of a CT scan or other radiographic procedure, it's possible that it may take a good part of a year to clear the stable iodine enough to avoid its interfering with the radioactive iodine. However, the length of time may vary from a couple of months to up to 10 months.

A method to determine when this iodine has cleared requires the following:

1) Follow the **LID** for one week. Maintain your usual thyroid hormone medication (note that this is not a preparation for scan or therapy).

2) On the last day of the diet, collect an accurate and full 24-hour urine specimen.

3) Have the urine sent for a total urine iodide analysis. A commercial laboratory that I've found to be reliable is at the Mayo Clinic in Rochester, MN.

4) A total urine iodide of 80 mcg (or less) in 24 hours demonstrates that the stable iodine interference has sufficiently passed to plan a radioactive iodine scan or therapy.

5) If the urine iodide is much higher, it may be useful to wait one to two months and repeat sequence 1) through 4) to evaluate the body's stable iodine content. This sequence is repeated until the urine value is sufficiently low. A urine iodide value that is sufficiently low demonstrates that the full scan or therapy preparation may be initiated without interference from the previous contrast dye administration. This is the general method I advise physicians to follow to determine when their patient may be sufficiently cleared of such stable iodine contamination. However, clinical situations may arise in which it isn't possible to wait until every parameter is optimal.

Are there other sources of stable iodine?

There are several sources of stable iodine that can block the uptake of radioactive iodine, despite carefully following a **LID** and avoiding contrast dye from CT scans. Iodine solutions may be used for douches or for cleansing skin wounds. It's also possible that lipsticks containing Red Dye #3 increase stable iodine. You may not be able to predict every potential stable iodine source; however, diligent efforts are likely to prove effective.

THE LOW IODINE CUPBOARD:

WHAT TO BUY AND HOW TO SHOP FOR THE LOW IODINE DIET

If you've read the Introduction, you'll see there are many specific restrictions for the Low Iodine Diet (LID), which include anything with iodized salt or dairy products. This chapter will help you shop for the food products you'll need to properly follow the LID. You'll also learn how to interpret the nutrition labels on your packaged food to determine whether they are "LID-safe."

The information in this chapter can be used in tandem with the Nutritional Analysis Chart in chapter 10. To make this chapter easy to understand, I want you to imagine that you are in a supermarket, and ready to do a large shopping trip. Get your cart. Now, let's walk through the aisles together, starting with the inside aisles, where we usually find the packaged food items, and finishing with the outside aisles, where we normally find our meats, produce, baked goods and so on.

PACKAGED FOOD IN THE INSIDE AISLES: WHAT'S OKAY, WHAT'S NOT

In the Introduction, Dr. Ain explains the importance of reading the labels on all packaged food items. To recap, the "no-no" ingredients in *packaged food items* you have to watch out for are:

- Iodized salt (unless it *specifies* "non-iodized salt"—don't buy it);
- Sea salt (frequently found in natural or organic food items);
- FD&C Red Dye # 3 (so, artificially red-colored foods, orange or even

purple foods with no dye listed in the ingredients are suspect, and should be avoided);

- Dried milk powders, found in most chocolate products and packaged baked items;
- Dried egg powders;
- Bread products that contain iodate dough conditioners (even salt-free bread could be baked with iodine dough conditioners, so just avoid. Also watch out for products containing breadcrumbs or dairy);
- Soy (no soy sauce or soy milk, or *soybean protein* products, such as tofu; soybean oil, often mixed with other vegetable oils or as an ingredient in vegetable shortening, is fine);
- Molasses (no brown sugar, and several other packaged items; sulfured molasses may be a high source of iodine, but since there is no reliable way to tell if molasses is sulfured or unsulfured, avoid all forms);
- Foods that contain the additives carragen, agar-agar, algin or alginates (these are seaweed or kelp by-products);
- Vitamins or food supplements with iodine; and
- Medications with iodine: Check with your doctor about which medications you can avoid and which medications you need to be on during the LID.

Look for "salt-free" versions of your favorite foods

Since so many people have to watch their blood pressure these days and must lower sodium in their diets, many packaged food items are now available in salt-free versions. Salt-free *does not* mean sodium-free, and foods with no salt can still have sodium (see the Nutrition Chart at the back of this book). Again, sodium is okay; salt is not okay! The list of salt-free products available is long, and getting longer, but commonly found items include:

- Canned tomatoes and tomato sauces;
- Canned vegetables and legumes of all kinds;
- Canned fruits (beware of fruit cocktails as the cherries have red dye!);

- A variety of soups (can be tricky, so read the labels carefully; or try some of the delicious soup recipes I've included in this book);
- Packaged crunchy snacks, such as corn chips, tortilla chips, and even some brands of potato chips (but be careful of soy protein products in salt-free crunchables, and do see my recipe for homemade potato chips on page 245, as well as the section entitled "Getting Creative with Non-iodized Salts" on page 242);
- Natural popcorn that you can make yourself;
- Nuts and dried fruits;
- Peanut butter;
- Many varieties of rice crackers, and
- Various brands of cold cereals (such as shredded wheat cereals or bran cereals).

Careful

"Natural flavorings" may include salt. Products that are unnaturally orange, red, pink, etc. may have food dyes that aren't allowed, even if the dyes aren't listed.

Finding Non-iodized Salt

If you live in the United States, you should be able to find non-iodized salt right beside the regular iodized salt. Additionally, several types of Kosher salts may come in non-iodized versions, but always check labels. If you live in Canada, only iodized salt is sold as "free-flowing" granulated salt. But you can still find Kosher salt, and again, check the label to ensure it is indeed *non-iodized* Kosher salt. You can salt many of your salt-free store-bought items on your own. For salt-free tortilla chips or other crunchy items, take your non-iodized salt and grind it up into a finer crystal. You can use a mortar and pestle, or put it in a plastic sandwich bag and run a rolling pin over it. A coffee grinder also works well. Take the finely ground salt, pour it into your snack bag, and just shake it up! You can freely add as much non-iodized salt as you wish to any of my recipes that say "non-iodized salt to taste." If you live outside of the United States or Canada, contact your local agricultural department or ministry and ask about what kinds of non-iodized

21

salts are available to consumers. And, see the section entitled "Getting Creative with Non-iodized Salts" on page 242.

Finding Commercial Bread Substitutes

Any *home-baked* bread is perfectly fine, and I have provided you with many good and easy bread recipes. But for those of you not interested in baking your own bread, the best bread substitute is a product I'm very familiar with: *Matzo*. Matzo is an unleavened bread product, made with just flour and water. It looks like a very flat waffle or large square cracker. It's widely available in most supermarkets (sometimes under International Foods), and comes in salt-free versions. One of the things I'm known for as a cookbook author is coming up with "bread substitute" recipes for Passover, a Jewish holiday that usually coincides with Easter (my Jewish readers need about 10-days worth of Passover recipes, a holiday in which all leavened bread products must be omitted). Actually, the "Last Supper" of Jesus was supposedly a Passover meal, at which he ate matzo. It's really lucky you ran into me! I've shared many of my bread-substitute recipes for you in this book.

For a breadcrumb substitute, and a great ingredient for baking all sorts of things year-round, *matzo meal* (ground matzo, which looks like a coarse flour) can be used. You can find this product right beside the matzo. Matzo meal is normally sold as salt-free, but double-check the labels. I have many recipes in this cookbook that use matzo meal. In fact, many people keep matzo meal handy all the time. You may also like a Jewish soup dumpling, called a *matzo ball*, so-named because it's made with matzo meal.

Other good bread substitutes are salt-free tortillas—either corn or flour. Again, please read labels to see if they contain salt. Whenever you see the term "LID-safe bread" in any of the recipes in this book, this term includes LID-safe tortillas.

Fats and Oils

All fats and oils, including soybean oil, are okay, and since butter and milk products are not allowed on the LID, you will need these to make foods taste good. Since many of you will be hypothyroid and will want to watch your cholesterol or prevent weight gain, and since some of you will need to watch these year-round, it's important to focus on the right fats and oils for your cooking needs. You generally want an oil that's monounsaturated—a "good fat." Luckily, the saturated fats from butter will be avoided during the LID.

Here's a good list of oils to buy for the LID, which are also *good for you*:

- Olive oil is always a great choice because it's 74 percent monounsaturated, which means it can actually lower cholesterol levels and protect against heart disease. You can use olive oil for just about everything; Mediterranean cooks even sprinkle it on bread in place of butter, and over pasta (with a little garlic) in place of fattier cream or tomato sauces. So, when dressing salads, olive oil is actually a far better bet than some of the "non-fat" options available today. As for baking, it used to be that olive oils were considered too strong. These days, however, there are many light olive oils on the market that boast a very neutral taste. So there's rarely, if ever, any need to stray from this "protective" cooking tool. In my baking recipes here, I still recommend canola oil.
- Other monounsaturated oils are canola, flaxseed, peanut, soybean, and avocado. Canola is second-in-line to olive oil, and is 50 percent monounsaturated. Canola oil is extracted from rapeseed, which comes from the cabbage family.
- Non-stick (and non-fat) cooking sprays are also fabulous for use in low-fat cooking because they completely eliminate the need for butter. These sprays also come in flavors like lemon and garlic, which add a whole lot of taste without the fat. If you coat your saucepan with cooking spray first, you'll only need to add a very small amount of oil for low-fat stir-fries and so on. In most cases, just a teaspoon is enough—especially with the flavored varieties, which pack a wallop of taste. As always, read your

labels to ensure that these products are completely SALT-FREE.

- For delicious low-fat marinades, fruit juice, garlic, and fresh ginger also add a ton of flavor and moisture without the fat. I have many recipes that incorporate these ingredients.

Pastas and Rice

If you don't care about the carbs, you can have as much pasta and rice as you like. Furthermore, you can have any kind of rice you wish; as Dr. Ain explains in his Introduction, there's no need to restrict rice intake. Filled pastas (such as tortellini or ravioli) typically have lots of salt or cheese, so *don't* choose these. Also, *you can't have egg-based pastas* (such as egg noodles). Whole wheat pastas are higher in fiber, and brown rice is higher in fiber than white pasta or white rice. Many pasta sauces in this cookbook will go beautifully with just plain pasta! And if you're on a low-carb diet, spaghetti squash, steamed spinach, broccoli or other cooked vegetables can substitute for pastas, rice, couscous or other starchy carbs normally eaten with sauces.

Beverages

The only beverages you can't have are beverages that contain salt (e.g., V-8, Bloody Mary mixes); seafood (e.g., Clamato juice); soy protein (e.g., soy milk); Red Dye # 3 (e.g., red or orange soft drinks); or dairy (milk, or other milk products, discussed more below). Cola, clear soft drinks (e.g., Sprite or sparkling waters), lemonade, etc. are fine. All natural juices with no added salt, coffee, tea, and so forth are allowed. For instant coffees, iced teas, etc., check labels carefully, but these are usually fine. Alcohol, such as beer and wine, etc., is allowed on the LID, but for those who are hypothyroid, it should be restricted or avoided *because the hypothyroid liver can't metabolize it well.* For these reasons, none of the recipes in this book require the use of wine or other alcohol. Please note also that cooking wine, which contains 1.5 percent salt to render it non-drinkable, must also be avoided.

FRESH FOODS: THE OUTSIDE AISLES

When shopping for the LID, the outside aisles will be your best bet! You can purchase all fruits and vegetables, no exceptions. And, yes—you can have rhubarb and potato skins (see Dr. Ain's Introduction). You'll especially want "rabbit food" on hand: carrot sticks and celery sticks make for great snacks, and I have many recipes for dips that are perfect for carrots and celery. A lot of the recipes in this cookbook use tomatoes. You can buy SALT-FREE canned tomatoes, or just use fresh tomatoes (I give you the option of either one in the recipes). Little cherry or grape tomatoes make great snacks, and sun-dried tomatoes are also terrific (just make sure they're UNSALTED)

To stock your fridge with the best fruits and veggies (especially if you're hypothyroid) choose:

- Fruits and veggies that are high in fiber. These include legumes, citrus fruit, strawberries, and apple pulp.
- Fruits and veggies that are high in vitamins A (and carotenoids), C, E, and potassium (for heart-healthy nutrients).

Meats

All fresh meats are fine, and you don't have to limit quantities for the LID specifically (although there may be other reasons to limit quantities—such as heart health, etc.). Some meats have broth injected into them: Turkey, chicken and pork are notorious when sold packaged. Just go to the butcher's counter and get them fresh. Usually the packages will disclose whether or not there is broth.

As an author of many low-fat cookbooks, I believe that lean meats are preferable for those of you who are watching your weight, or are hypothyroid. Since meat is a key player when it comes to fat in the diet, and you can't have any fish or seafood, choose from:

- Lean beef (round, sirloin, chuck, or loin). Look for "choice" or "select" grades instead of "prime," and lean or extra-lean ground beef (with no more than 15 percent fat).
- Lean veal, pork (tenderloin, loin chop) and lean lamb (leg, arm, or loin).
- Chicken, Cornish hen, and turkey (all without skins). You can also substitute ground turkey for ground beef in burgers.
- Chicken breast or drumstick instead of chicken wing or thigh.
- Exotic meats, such as emu, buffalo, rabbit, pheasant, and venison. These have less total fat than animals commonly raised for market.

Dairy Case Woes

The only things you can buy in the dairy case are eggs, as you *can* have egg whites. You may also find egg whites in a carton (make sure they're pure with no funny additives). Egg substitutes should be avoided, as they usually contain some yolk product.

What about margarine? *Most brands of margarine can't be used on the LID* due to a common ingredient: sodium caseinate (a milk protein derivative that hasn't yet been evaluated for iodine content). In addition, many margarines (even if they are salt-free) contain milk solids or soy protein. Sodium caseinate remains untested with respect to iodine content, so it should be avoided. If you *can* find margarines without sodium caseinate or milk solids that are salt-free, then that's fine. The LID-safe margarine I've identified as of writing this is Fleischmann's SALT-FREE and DAIRY-FREE margarine, which you can find in most supermarkets in larger urban centers. To accommodate those of you who can't find this margarine, none of the recipes in this book require margarine (or butter), with only one exception (a shortbread cookie you can make with LID-safe margarine). I also provide information on baking substitutes in the Desserts chapter, in case you do find a LID-safe margarine.

There are other unhealthy things about margarine due to the process of hydrogenation, which is what turns it into a "spreadable" butter-like product and creates trans fats, which, experts warn, should be avoided.

You can use shortening or lard for baking recipes that normally call for butter or margarine, too.

Milk Substitutes

Sadly, no milk, or cheeses, or any other dairy products are allowed on the LID. Soy milk and soy cheese products are also not allowed. I provide several delicious milk substitutes in chapter 4, such as rice milk, almond milk and coconut milk, as well as ways to have these as chocolate milks. Store-bought rice milk has SEA SALT so you'll need to make this yourself. Some store-bought nut milk brands contain no salt (there are several brands of coconut milk that should be fine) but read the labels; they're few and far between.

Baked Goods: Keep on Walking!

Again, commercially baked goods usually have iodine from the machinery used to bake them, or from salt, which is frequently not labeled. Bake your own baked goods; there are many recipes in this book. Or, substitute SALT-FREE matzo and rice crackers for breads, or use other LID-safe products. If you live in a smaller community, you may be able find a local bakery that can guarantee LID-safe baked goods as well.

Bulk Food Bins

You can choose from most of the items normally found in bulk food bins, unless they contain salt. The whole grains and beans that you'll find in the bulk food bins may even be the best places to find salt-free alternatives to the canned beans you normally buy. Bulk food items are generally more affordable than the processed or packaged variety you may be used to eating. They're also high-fiber items, which you'll want if you're hypothyroid. And when properly stored, they last forever! When preparing for the LID, look for the following:

- Dried beans and peas (great for soups and stews).
- Rolled oat flakes instead of packaged or "instant" cereal.
- Barley, for use in soups (as well as on its own). Also high in fiber.
- Rice and pastas. In general, it's always a good idea to opt for those grains that have undergone the least amount of processing.
- Whole grains—such as bulgur, couscous—as another alternative to breads or a common white starch. Both of these grains, when added to vegetables, can transform a healthy starch into a hearty meal.
- Unsalted, natural peanut butter.

STOCKING UP ON SNACK FOODS

In this book, I devote a whole chapter to snacks, and provide a list of many packaged goods you can buy, in addition to dozens of snack foods you can make. Check out chapter 8!

STORING AND FREEZING

If you're going to be hypothyroid while you're on a LID, it's important to plan your LID cupboard in advance. Set aside one cupboard for all your canned and packaged items. Put your non-iodized salt into a different salt shaker so you don't confuse it, or just keep the box handy. If you're using non-iodized Kosher salt, you may need to grind it.

Next, in your freezer, set aside a shelf for all your frozen items, including the recipes you've made in advance, such as sauces, soups, stews, etc. Then when you're on the diet, it's easier for you to just grab items from the LID freezer shelf, thaw and eat. Make sure you label things clearly if you are planning to be hypothyroid.

FREEZE-AHEAD RECIPES

Many of the recipes in this book can be made ahead of time and frozen, including baked goods, sauces, soups, stews, meat dishes, vegetable dishes, etc. I encourage you to do this if you're going to be hypothyroid, so that you don't have to worry about cooking when you're not feeling up to it. Let this book be the Mom that comes to visit and leaves you meals in the freezer that you just thaw. For those of you who aren't hypothyroid, enjoy this cookbook as you would any other. I've made everything easy and delicious!

IF YOU'RE ON ANOTHER DIET, TOO

Many of you who must go on the LID are on other diets for health reasons. Here are some guidelines for the various types of diets many of us are on.

Low-Fat, or Heart Healthy

No problem—this really is the book for you. There's nothing in this book you can't have, and many of the baking recipes are lower in fat and cholesterol, and higher in fiber, than their originals. Many of these recipes will be terrific year-round, or when you're not on the LID. If you're also watching your sodium, simply adjust the amounts of non-iodized salt. And, use the Nutritional Analysis Chart in chapter 10 to help you count calories, fats, etc.

Low-Carb or Carb Counting

There are plenty of recipes in this book to suit the low-carb eater, or the person with diabetes who's forced to keep an eye on carb intake. Stick to the meats and vegetables, and use pasta substitutes, such as cooked spinach or other greens, spaghetti squash, etc. Lean chicken breasts are also great substitutes for pastas, which you can put pasta sauces on. The milk substitutes are actually excellent for the low-carb dieter, too. For the breakfasts, they'll be more suitable than the fare you'd normally find—particularly the pancake recipes! Again, use the Nutritional Analysis Chart in chapter 10 to help you count carbs.

Lactose-Intolerant or Dairy-Free

Nothing in this book will be a problem for you, since all dairy is omitted. For those of you who require dairy-free recipes (e.g., those who are Kosher, vegan, and so on), you'll find dozens of dairy-free or pareve recipes that can be used instead of your alternatives year-round. Enjoy.

The Gluten-Free Diet

Those of you living with celiac disease or wheat allergies will find the challenges of gluten-free living similar to those of the LID. You'll find that your success and ease with both diets is based on two very straightforward principles:

1. Choosing foods that are simple and fresh rather than packaged or processed.
2. Avoiding any foods that you can't confirm are safe.

Gluten is the protein found in wheat. But gluten has been modified and used in many different ways by the processed food industry. As a result, celiac associations differ in their guidelines about what the gluten-free diet should and should not contain. All agree, however, that the following foods must be avoided: wheat, rye, barley, spelt, oats, kamut and triticale.

Contact your local celiac association to familiarize yourself with the basics of the gluten-free diet.

CHAPTER TWO

LID MEAL PLANNING: A SAMPLE LID MENU

The three-day menu that follows is a sample of an ideal low iodine diet. It is only meant as an example; there are limitless combinations and choices that can make your daily menus varied and appealing! This plan is based on the recipes in this book, which begin in Part 2. All of the recipes in this chapter can be found on the page numbers indicated.

DAY ONE
Breakfast
Basic Savory Egg White Omelet (see page 59)
with optional asparagus, broccoli, spinach, tomatoes, Italian herbs, tomato sauce or hot sauce, and *Low Iodine Ketchup* (see page 183)
Dill Onion Bread (see page 68)

Mid-Morning Snack
Baked Apple (see page 227)
or a whole fresh apple or orange

Lunch
Luscious Lentil Soup (see page 131)
Unique and Yummy Vegetable Salad (see page 95)

Mid-Afternoon Snack
Matzo-Style Flatbread (see page 247) with *Smoky Eggplant Dip* (see page 256)
or *Avocado Guacamole* (see page 249)

Dinner
Old-Fashioned Hamburgers (see page 115)
Yum-Yum Potato Wedgies (see page 101)
Honey-Glazed Carrots (see page 140)

Dessert (Optional)
Basically Great Apple Pie (see page 215)

Beverages
Breakfasts: Juice, coffee or tea with milk substitutes (see page 49)
various milk substitutes or shakes (see page 49)
Lunch or Dinner or throughout the day: Herbal tea, mineral water,
fruit juice and clear sodas throughout the day as desired, so
long as sodas do not contain red food coloring.

DAY TWO
Breakfast
Quick-Cooking Oatmeal (see page 48)
with optional raisins, chopped dates or apricots
No-Knead Cinnamon Coffee Cake (see page 72)
one whole grapefruit

Mid-Morning Snack
Pumpkin Seeds (see page 258)

Lunch
Noodle Bake (see page 104)
Tomato, Onion, and Pepper Salad (see page 94)

Mid-Afternoon Snack
Crisp Lasagna Chips (see page 244)
with *Super Salsa* (see page 257)
or one cup fresh carrot sticks

Dinner
Veal Normande (see page 178)
Grilled Lyonnaise Potatoes (see page 99)
Apricot Candied Carrots (see page 138)

Dessert (Optional)
Dried Fruit Compote (see page 227)

DAY THREE
Breakfast
Carrots-for-Breakfast Pancakes (see page 62)
Homemade Applesauce (see page 228)

Mid-Morning Snack
Best Blueberry Orange Muffins (see page 66)
or one fresh banana

Lunch
Garden Vegetable Soup (see page 127)
Cabbage Rolls (see page 110)

Mid-Afternoon Snack
Tomato and Basil Bruschetta (see page 259)
or *Roasted Red Peppers* (see page 259)

Dinner

Herb Roasted Chicken (see page 155)
Basic Polenta (see page 46)
Mixed Green Salad with Orange Balsamic Vinaigrette (see page 93)

Dessert (Optional)

Lemon Loaf (see page 210)

CHAPTER THREE

LID ON THE TOWN

It's difficult to expect people on a LID to behave like "shut-ins" for two weeks, and not venture out at all. In addition, many people on the LID will find themselves in restaurants for business or social reasons that are unavoidable. Some people want to go out for anniversaries or birthdays, and they may be on the LID during these special occasions. This chapter is designed to address the question: *What should I do when I have to eat out?* In a world of life-threatening food allergies and dozens of special health diets (including many salt-free diets for people with hypertension), restaurants have learned to accommodate us, and most, if not all, will adjust.

It's important to remember that you can never know *for sure* what's in your food unless you're cooking it yourself, but there has to be some level of trust in a good restaurant with a responsible manager and chef. If you can't trust the restaurant, or can't relax enough to know that the food is safe, then *don't* dine out, or just don't order anything other than a fruit plate, etc.

But if dining out is unavoidable, or simply something you really want, then this chapter is for you.

THE FIRST STEPS

The hospitality industry isn't called the *hospitality* industry for nothing, and these days, dealing with food restrictions is just one component of good service. Consider taking your first steps in a favorite neighborhood or restaurant district. Most establishments post menus outside, and a quick glance at the night's offerings will often confirm whether or not you'll find something that's LID-safe. Once you become familiar with the ingredients that are off-limits to the LID diner, you'll get to know where these ingredients crop up in various cuisines.

You'll then be able to tell at a glance which items on a menu can be altered to suit your needs, and which you'll want to avoid altogether.

If friends or colleagues have chosen the restaurant for you, consider calling in advance (ideally during off hours) to get a sense of the menu. Why not toss your non-iodized salt and homemade tomato sauce or salad dressing into your briefcase or purse and then work on your conversational skills over the phone—you'll need them later!

STARTERS

Simpler, fresher choices are best, as they're often much easier to dissect. Choose a salad and request, if you can't confirm that the dressing is safe, a bottle each of olive oil and balsamic vinegar. Some restaurants (particularly Italian) will bring these condiments to your table alongside the dinner rolls or bread; and almost all restaurants will have them on hand in the kitchen.

Soups are rarely made to order and are not good choices. Puréed soups are more common these days than cream-based soups, but even these healthier options are typically made with salt, as are clear soups and broth.

Grilled veggies (or some variation thereof) are a popular item on many of today's menus. They are typically made with olive oil, not butter, and are a great choice for the LID diner. You must give instructions in advance to *not* salt while preparing. As always, confirm with staff on this, and on repeat visits (oftentimes a recipe can vary depending on who's preparing it), that everything you've chosen is safe.

MAINS

Entrées tend to combine food groups, which means it will be more important than ever to *ask questions*. Once you've eliminated the more obvious choices (such as seafood or cheese manicotti) you can turn your attention to some possible LID pitfalls. Sauces can be tricky, as they're often prepared in advance with salt, molasses, soy, or even sea products (e.g., oyster sauce). Stuffed dishes (such as stuffed chicken) are typically prestuffed with breadcrumbs. And anything that's pan-fried (such as chicken, and some pastas) *might* have been prepared with butter.

If the entrée you want comes with butter roasted potatoes, take a look at the other available mains. Why not substitute those potatoes for a baked potato, extra salad or veggies? Most kitchens, particularly busy kitchens, prefer substitutions to out-and-out requests for a personal chef.

Finally, if the dish you took the trouble to dissect and then order arrives looking suspicious *in any way*, don't hesitate to visit the kitchen. A *friendly* request for confirmation that your needs were understood, and that your order is safe, is your right. Just remember to say thank-you as well!

DESSERTS

Steer clear of commercially prepared baked goods (i.e., anything made at outside bakeries or cake shops), as their ingredients are hard to verify. Otherwise, you'll want to avoid the usual suspects: dairy and eggs. Sadly, this cancels out most pies, crumbles, pastries and cakes. Be aware too that even sweet things are sometimes made with salt. And check for sneaky ingredients like molasses and breadcrumbs.

If this feels futile, it isn't. There are plenty of desserts (like gelatos, and stewed or poached fruit) that are just as tasty, and healthier to boot. On a slow night, consider asking the kitchen to whip you up a LID-safe surprise. Or, bring your own cookies (see the Desserts chapter) or dark, non-dairy chocolate (see page 244 for more information on what chocolates you *can* eat), and watch as other customers envy *you!*

MAKE IT OFFICIAL

Use the following letter to help you clarify just what you can and can't eat when dining out. After photocopying it, keep a stack of "extras" stashed in your purse, or in the glove compartment of your car, to help get your needs met at nearly every restaurant in town.

Dear Restaurant Manager:

For health reasons, I am on a LOW IODINE DIET. This means that I MUST NOT eat anything prepared with salt (iodized and sea salt), dairy (including yogurt and butter), seafood or sea products (including fish sauce), soy or soy products (including tofu), Red Dye #3 (often a component of red, red-orange or brown food coloring), molasses or eggs (whites are okay).

Even the smallest amount of any one of these can affect my health. Please avoid serving me anything that contains the above ingredients, as well as any sauces, dressings or breads (including breadcrumbs) that contain them.

Your attention and assistance in providing me with a SAFE meal is greatly appreciated. The ingredients to avoid are:

- Salt
- Dairy (including butter)
- Molasses
- Seafood or sea products
- Soy or soy products
- Egg yolks

LID AROUND THE WORLD

Thanks to today's global village, eating out is a multicultural experience. Once reserved for the urbanites among us, ethnic diversity is now as close as the nearest town or strip mall—where you'd be hard pressed *not* to find at least one Chinese restaurant. But how much you have to choose from will naturally depend on your neighborhood, so it's best to familiarize yourself in advance with the challenges of a multicultural menu.

This time you may encounter a language barrier: For this reason, there are more problems with some international cuisines that are outlined here.

Problems with Chinese and Vietnamese Restaurants

Your biggest challenge with these common Asian options is avoiding the soy sauce that accompanies many of the meat and vegetable dishes. Dark sauce (hoisin) must also be avoided, as must fish (oyster) sauce or anything made with molasses. To navigate in Asian restaurants:

- Avoid them if possible.
- Kindly inform the kitchen of your food restrictions, especially with respect to salt, eggs, molasses, and soy (many dishes actually serve soy on the side, and are therefore LID-safe).
- Avoid tofu—it's a soy product and may contain dangerous iodine levels.
- Opt out of the buffet entirely.
- Avoid egg noodles.
- Avoid rice, as it's often cooked in salt.
- Bring your own non-iodized salt.

If you're stuck, order dishes that are made on the spot with fresh ingredients, such as a vegetable stir-fry or a meat dish. Garlic and herbs are okay, but ask that no salt be used in preparation. Request that all sauces be omitted and, after first asking your dining partner to taste what you order for salt, just salt the food yourself for taste with your own non-iodized salt.

Problems with Greek Restaurants

The biggest culprits here are dairy and seafood. That means, sadly, no flaming cheeses or fried calamari for you! Fortunately, Greek fare offers alternatives for the LID diner, including delicious souvlaki dinners (minus the salt, tzatziki and butter) as well as many tasty vegetable options. When in Greek town:

- Kindly inform the kitchen of your food restrictions.
- Consider a Greek salad without the feta. This is a delicious, healthy option (so long as you confirm that the dressing accompanying it is safe—or, better yet, bring your own from home).
- Remember that tzatziki (the white dressing or dip that's served as a side with much of Greek fare) is made with yogurt and must therefore be avoided.
- Make sure that any other pre-made offerings (such as hummus, babaghanouj, tapanades and grape leaves) are salt and dairy-free. Sometimes they can be made fresh.
- Check that the rice and potatoes (which come with most meals) are free of butter and salt; if you can't verify this, ask for vegetables, a baked potato, or salad.
- Don't forget your non-iodized salt.

Problems with Indian Restaurants

Indian food is wonderfully varied, but much of it's served in the form of stews or curries. Even the delicious sides or snacks (fried vegetable pakoras, for example, or the flat, cracker-like breads called papadum) are often prepared in advance. This makes LID dining especially challenging. Unless your server can assure you that a particular dish is LID-safe, it's best to steer clear of these pre-pared foods. Opt instead for dishes over which you can exert some control. Additionally:

- Make sure your naan wasn't fried in butter.
- Pay special attention to sneaky LID pitfalls with respect to dairy (for

example, Indian cuisine commonly uses yogurt for its cooling properties).

- Avoid gulping down a lassi, India's favorite yogurt drink.
- Be aware that many Indian desserts are made with milk.
- Bring along your own non-iodized salt.
- Inform the kitchen of your food restrictions, as always.

Problems with Japanese Restaurants

If you find yourself in a Japanese restaurant, accept the fact that it's about the worst place to be when you're on the LID. Request a meat dish prepared on the spot with no salt or sauces used, and see if you can get a fresh salad (you can use your own dressing, or ask for some sesame oil). Soy or teriyaki sauces are common culprits. You might also opt for vegetable tempura, if you can verify that the batter is made with no unsafe ingredients. Also, stay away from tofu, which is a soy product.

Sushi, of course, is about the worst thing you can have on a LID diet. If the fish isn't a dead giveaway, consider also the seaweed wrapper. Called nori, this seaweed by-product is very high in iodine (as are all foods that contain additives such as carrageen, agar-agar, algin, and alginate, which are made from seaweed by-products).

All the rice is usually pre-made and prepared with salt, so stay away, unless you can be assured that it was freshly steamed with no salt. As always, inform the kitchen of your food restrictions and work with staff to see if there's anything in the restaurant you can have.

Problems with Italian Restaurants

All pasta can be made fresh, just for you, without salted water. You can request the pasta be made with just an olive oil and garlic sauce, with no salt, and then add your own. Alternatively, a little advance planning and a few ounces of homemade tomato sauce (see recipes, page 189 and 192) will go a long way towards making your Italian dining experience an enjoyable one. You'll need to avoid any cheesy dishes (pizzas and pastas made with cheese, or antipasto plates in which cheese figures prominently) but all other pastas make good dinner options. Inform staff of your diet restrictions so they know not to use salted water, or serve you a pasta made with egg noodles. Choose a fresh salad as a starter, then dress your pasta of choice with the delicious sauce you've brought from home, as well as your own non-iodized salt.

Be aware, however, that there are some sneaky LID pitfalls in traditional Italian fare. They are:

- Breadcrumbs. Many Italian recipes ask for breadcrumbs, so be diligent with your server.
- Parmesan. This cheese is harder to detect, and it's particularly common in pastas and risottos.
- Milk or cream. Cream is often a component of Italian risottos; it's even more often a part of Italian desserts. Request that the kitchen prepare your risotto without butter or cream, and opt for gelato or fresh fruit for dessert.

Problems with Latin and Mexican Restaurants

The biggest culprits here are cheese and seafood, but you'll also need to ensure that any dishes containing guacamole, refried beans or salsa are salt-free. Tortillas (the popular Mexican flatbreads made with corn or wheat) are fine, so long as they're made without salt, and ask about whether eggs are used in any dishes, too. Inform staff of your diet restrictions at the outset, and have your server clarify for you which items on the menu are LID-safe. Spanish and Cuban restaurants often feature a "tapas" menu. This is a real treat for anyone with food restrictions, as it tends to mean lots of choice (the portions are tiny) and few surprises.

Problems with Thai Restaurants

Thai food is both sweet and savory, simple and complex. And the great thing about it? Much of it is LID-safe. Most Thai dishes are rice- or rice noodle-based, and are made fresh. You can request that they also be made *without* salted water. Cold rice paper rolls are a delicious choice for a starter, as they're made with crunchy fresh vegetables, coriander and rice noodles, and the dipping sauce is on the side. The rice paper rolls are usually unsalted, but double-check just to be sure. Traditional pad Thai is a good bet for a main, but make sure it's prepared without eggs, tofu, or salty fermented fish sauce (*nam pla* or *nuoc nam*). You'll typically encounter problems with the sauces, which are often prepared in advance. So, ask for a list of dishes made on the spot, and then review your options. As always, tuck your LID letter into your pocket next to your non-iodized salt. And kindly inform staff of your food restrictions at the beginning of the meal.

Other things to watch out for include:

- Fish sauce (*nam pla*). This is used extensively in Thai cooking, so you'll need to inform staff that it must be avoided.
- Dipping sauces. These accompany many of the appetizers. Ask your server how each has been prepared.
- Tofu. This is easy to omit from recipes that include it.

Problems with Fast Food

Try the drive thru at fast food outlets, but there's absolutely no guarantee you'll find LID-safe fast foods, other than salads. Fast food outlets are not designed to accommodate special diets, and you'll need to stick to items you can verify are safe, such as a salad with no dressing, a baked potato (like you'd find at Wendy's) with nothing on it, and so on. If it has to be processed in some way, don't eat it. Even the normally safe sodas are often served up fast from tap, and can have dyes in them you wouldn't otherwise suspect. Get a salad and a bottled water.

BREAKFASTS
THE TOUGHEST MEALS

■ CEREALS

Basic Polenta (Cornmeal Mush or Grits)

4 cups water
1 tsp non-iodized salt
1 cup yellow or white cornmeal

1. Combine water and non-iodized salt in a large heavy saucepan and bring to a boil. Add cornmeal in a thin stream (like falling rain), stirring constantly. Reduce heat and cook over low heat for 20 minutes, stirring constantly with a long-handled spoon. Mixture will become a thick mass and pull away from the sides of the pan. For best results and lump-free polenta, don't stop stirring polenta until it is done.

Yield: 4 to 6 servings. Leftover polenta can be used to make meals for lunch or dinner, such as Grilled Polenta Wedges (below).

Leftover Polenta for Lunch or Dinner:
- *Top with lots of fried onions and/or mushrooms. Also delicious with gravy from roasted brisket or stew.*
- *Some people do a thicker version made in the microwave. They cook ¼ cup cornmeal with 1 cup water and a dash of salt (use non-iodized salt) in a 4 cup glass measure. Microwave covered on HIGH for 5 minutes, stirring at half time.*

Grilled Polenta Wedges: *Spread polenta evenly in a sprayed 9-inch pie plate. Chill for at least 2 hours, or until firm. Cut into wedges. Broil or grill wedges for 2 to 3 minutes per side until piping hot. Serve as appetizers or as a side starch.*

Polenta Pizza: *Pour hot polenta into a sprayed 9-inch round oven-proof casserole. Spread evenly. Top with sliced tomatoes, mushrooms, green and/or red peppers and garlic slivers. Drizzle lightly with olive oil. Season with pepper and basil. Bake uncovered at 350°F for 15 to 20 minutes. Cut in wedges.*

Cream of Wheat

For one serving, use ¼ cup cream of wheat and 1 cup tap water or apple juice. Combine in a microsafe bowl that holds at least twice the volume. Microwave uncovered on HIGH for 2 ½ to 3 minutes, stirring twice. Let stand for 1 minute. Cream of Wheat is delicious sweetened with honey or maple syrup. Or try it with applesauce, raisins, dried apricots (or any dried fruit), sliced fresh fruit, chopped unsalted nuts, or granola. Serve with Almond Milk (see page 50) or Rice Milk (see page 56).

Great Granola

Easier to make and healthier (not to mention salt-free!) than the commercial brands. Eat plain with no milk, or mix with Homemade Applesauce (see recipe, page 228), Almond Milk (see page 50), Rice Milk (see page 56), or apple juice. This also makes a great snack.

> ¼ cup oil
> ¾ cup honey
> ¼ cup maple syrup
> 3 cups quick-cooking oats or oat bran, or a combination of both
> ½ cup shredded coconut, optional
> 2 tbsp wheat germ, optional
> ½ cup sesame seeds
> ¾ cup chopped, unsalted nuts (pecans, filberts, walnuts, or almonds)
> 1 tsp cinnamon
> 1 tsp vanilla
> ½ cup raisins

1. Preheat oven to 350ºF.
2. Combine oil, honey, and maple syrup in a large bowl. Add remaining ingredients, except raisins, and mix well. Spread mixture on a large rimmed baking sheet. Bake uncovered for 30 to 35 minutes, or until toasted, stirring occasionally.
3. Stir in raisins. Let cool, stirring with a fork occasionally to break up mixture. Store in an airtight container in a cool, dry place.

Yield: About 6 cups. Can also be frozen.

Oat Bran Cereal

For 1 serving, measure ¼ cup oat bran cereal into a microsafe bowl (about 20 oz capacity). Add ¾ cup tap water. Microwave uncovered on HIGH for 1 minute, then on MEDIUM-LOW (30%) for 2 minutes.

Old-Fashioned Oatmeal

> 3 cups hot water
> ½ tsp non-iodized salt
> 1 ⅓ cups large flake oatmeal

1. Combine hot water, salt and oatmeal in a 3-quart microsafe casserole. Microwave uncovered on HIGH for 8 to 9 minutes, stirring at half time. Stir and let stand for 3 minutes.

Yield: 4 servings. Reheats well.

Quick-Cooking Oatmeal

Make sure to use a large enough cooking container as cereal boils over very easily. No sticking, no scorching—what a pleasure!

> ¼ cup quick-cooking oatmeal
> ½ cup water or apple juice

pinch of non-iodized salt
2 tsp honey or maple syrup
Almond Milk or Rice Milk (see page 50 and page 56)

1. Combine oatmeal, water and salt in a 16 oz microsafe bowl. Microwave
    uncovered on HIGH for 1 ½ minutes, until bubbling, stirring once. Or
    microwave uncovered on HIGH for 1 minute, then on MEDIUM-LOW
    (30%) for 1 minute for less chance of boil-over. Let stand for 1 minute.
2. Add Almond Milk (see page 50) or Rice Milk (see page 56) and honey or
    maple syrup. If desired, microwave uncovered on HIGH for 20 seconds
    longer. (I like my porridge hot!)

Yield: 1 serving.

Variations:
*   *If desired, add 2 tbsp raisins, chopped dates or apricots, and a sprinkling of
    cinnamon at the beginning of Step 2.*
*   *For 4 servings, use 1 cup oatmeal plus 2 cups water or apple juice. Use a 2- or
    3-quart microwavable casserole. Microwave uncovered on HIGH for 4 to 5
    minutes until thick, stirring halfway through cooking time. Stir and let stand
    for 2 to 3 minutes.*
*   *If you don't like your oatmeal as thick, use up to ¾ cup liquid for each
    ¼ cup of oatmeal. For 4 servings, use 1 cup oatmeal plus 2 ½ to 3 cups
    water or apple juice.*

■ MILK SUBSTITUTES, SMOOTHIES, AND SHAKES

In many cases, you can just add water to a recipe that asks for milk (especially
if it only requires minimal amounts). For coffee or tea, consider using 20 miniature marshmallows, which willl melt slowly and add a creamy texture. For cereals, try adding apple juice, or a banana puréed in some apple juice or water (also
a good replacement for yogurt). Or, consider the following milk substitutes.

Almond Banana Milk

 1 cup Almond Milk (see below)
 1 medium banana, peeled and cut in chunks

1.   Combine together in a blender or food processor and blend until creamy.
     Serve immediately.

Yield: 1 or 2 servings.

Variation: *Substitute Rice Milk (see page 56) for Almond Milk if you're allergic to almonds.*

Almond Fruit Shake

Add any of the following fresh or frozen fruits (or a combination of 1 cup
assorted fruits) to the Banana Shake recipe (see page 52), and blend together
until thick and creamy: 6 to 8 large strawberries; 1 large peach, nectarine or
mango (peeled, pitted, and cut in chunks). If desired, add a little maple syrup
or honey.

Almond Milk

Almond Milk makes a scrumptious substitute for regular milk in coffee or tea
and is very high in calcium. Add it to your breakfast cereal or use it in shakes
and smoothies. It can replace regular milk in baking recipes. When making soup
or sauces, always add the Almond Milk at the end of cooking and heat it gently.
Don't let it boil, as it has a tendency to break down.

 ½ cup blanched unsalted almonds (see page 51)
 1 tbsp maple syrup
 2 cups cold water

1.   In a large food processor or blender, grind nuts until fine, about 20 to 25
     seconds. (Don't overprocess or you'll get nut butter!) Add maple syrup to

water and stir to dissolve. While machine is running, slowly add water through the feed tube of the processor or the opening of the blender lid. Process for 2 minutes, until well blended.

2. Place a fine strainer over a large bowl. For a smoother texture, line strainer with cheesecloth or a paper coffee filter. Slowly pour Almond Milk into strainer and let it drain through. To speed up the draining process, stir it a few times, pressing down on the almonds with the back of a spoon.

3. Store Almond Milk in a covered jar or pitcher in the refrigerator. Stir before using. Store almond pulp in a separate container; refrigerate or freeze.

Yield: about 2 cups Almond Milk and ⅓ cup ground almond pulp. Keeps 4 to 5 days in the refrigerator.

Variations:
- *To blanch almonds: Place almonds in a bowl and cover completely with boiling water. Let stand for 5 to 10 minutes, until water has cooled down somewhat. Drain; peel off skins and discard. (Rubbing the almonds between paper towels makes this task easier.) Dry nuts before grinding.*
- *The ratio of water to nuts will determine the thickness of the nut milk. For a thicker mixture, use less water. This will produce a perfect replacement for heavy cream to pour over your favorite berries.*
- *Leftover almond pulp makes a delicious, fiber-rich addition to cereal or smoothies. Some people even like to use it as a facial scrub!*
- *Buy almonds in bulk for maximum freshness and minimum cost. Store almonds (or any nuts) in the freezer or refrigerator to prevent them from becoming rancid. One pound of almonds yields about 4 cups.*

Almond Strawberry Milk

Follow the recipe for Almond Banana Milk, but substitute 6 or 8 large, ripe strawberries for the banana.

Apple Banana Milk

½ cup Almond Milk (see page 50) or Rice Milk (see page 56)
½ cup apple juice
½ medium banana, peeled and cut in chunks
dash of cinnamon

1. Combine all ingredients together in a blender or food processor and blend until creamy. Serve immediately.

Yield: 1 serving.

Banana Shake

Freezing bananas makes a thick, creamy mixture that you can eat with a spoon! Place ripe bananas in a plastic freezer bag and store in the freezer—no need to peel them first. When required, remove them from the freezer and place under running water for 10 seconds. They'll be very easy to peel using a sharp knife.

1 ½ cups Almond Milk (see page 50) or Rice Milk (see page 56)
2 frozen medium bananas, peeled and cut in chunks (about 1 cup)

1. Combine ingredients together in a blender or food processor and blend until thick and creamy. Serve immediately.

Yield: 2 servings.

Cashew Milk

Follow the recipe for Almond Milk (see page 50), but substitute unsalted cashews for almonds. For a thicker liquid the consistency of heavy cream, just use less water—pour it over berries for a delicious treat. Cashew Milk makes an excellent alternative to coconut milk in curries and doesn't contain the saturated fat of coconut.

Chocolate Banana Shake

Follow the recipe for Banana Shake (on the previous page) but add 2 tbsp Chocolate Syrup (see page 55).

Cocoa-Nut Cocoa

You'll go co-co co-co-nuts over this delicious hot drink! If preparing with homemade coconut milk made from sweetened coconut, you won't need to add white sugar—it'll be sweet enough as is.

    1 tsp unsweetened pure cocoa powder (LID-safe)
    ¼ cup boiling water
    ¾ cup coconut milk (homemade or SALT-FREE canned)
    dash of vanilla extract
    white sugar to taste, if needed

1. Dissolve pure cocoa powder in boiling water. Stir in coconut milk and vanilla; mix well. Sweeten to taste. Microwave on HIGH for 45 to 60 seconds. Serve immediately.

Yield: 1 serving.

Coconut Milk

Several brands of canned coconut milk contain salt. If you're feeling ambitious, here's a "grate" way to make it yourself, including a quick variation. (The milky liquid inside the coconut is NOT coconut milk.)

    1 coconut
    hot water (as needed)

1. Pierce three holes at the peak of the coconut using a hammer and nail. Drain out liquid. Place coconut in a 400ºF oven for 15 to 20 minutes. Remove from oven and let cool until you're able to handle it comfortably.

2. Wrap in a heavy towel and crack the shell by tapping it with a hammer. Have a bowl handy to catch the milky liquid. Peel off inner brown skin with a potato peeler. Rinse coconut, pat dry with paper towels and cut in chunks.

3. Process 1 to 1 ½ cups at a time on the Steel Blade of your food processor, using on/off pulses, then let the machine run until finely ground, about 20 seconds longer. (Or chop in the blender, no more than ½ cup at a time.)

4. To prepare coconut milk, pour hot water over coconut. (For each cup of coconut, add 1 cup of water.) Let stand 5 minutes, then process or blend for 1 to 2 minutes, until milky. Drain through a double layer of cheesecloth. (A Donvier yogurt strainer also works well.) Squeeze or press the coconut pulp until quite dry.

5. Refrigerate the drained liquid (coconut milk). Stir before using.

Yield: 1 cup grated coconut plus water yields 1 cup coconut milk. It will keep for 3 or 4 days in the refrigerator.

Chef's Tips:
- **Quick Coconut Milk:** *Instead of fresh coconut, substitute packaged unsweetened shredded coconut. Check package labels carefully—some brands contain salt and some are very sweet. Follow directions above, beginning with Step 4.*
- *A medium coconut yields 4 to 5 cups grated coconut.*
- *Use equal amounts of grated coconut and hot water to make coconut milk. Some people like to use the natural milky coconut liquid plus hot water as the liquid.*
- *Leftover coconut pulp can be refrigerated or frozen. Add it to cake, muffin or cookie batters.*
- *Coconut milk is sensitive to high heat, so add it to hot sauces or foods at the last minute (or cook it over hot water). Coconut milk can be used in coffee, tea, or cereal as a milk substitute.*

Dairy-Free Smoothie

If both the banana and strawberries are frozen, you'll get a thicker smoothie.

> 1 frozen banana, cut in chunks
> 1 cup strawberries (fresh or frozen)
> 1 cup apple or orange juice

1. Combine all ingredients in a blender or food processor and blend until thick and creamy. Serve immediately.

Yield: 1 to 2 servings.

Variations: *Instead of strawberries, substitute peeled peaches, nectarines, mango, papaya, or pineapple, cut in chunks. Use cranberry or pineapple juice as the liquid. For natural sweetness and a flavor boost, add 2 or 3 large pitted dates.*

Easy Chocolate Syrup

Delicious added to smoothies, shakes, Almond Milk (see page 50) or Rice Milk (see page 56).

> 1 cup unsweetened pure cocoa powder (LID-safe)
> 2 cups white sugar
> 1 ¾ cups cold water
> 1 tsp vanilla extract, if desired

1. Combine cocoa and sugar in a saucepan; gradually whisk in water. Heat on medium heat until simmering. Reduce heat and continue to cook until smooth and thick, whisking constantly, for about 5 minutes.
2. Let cool; stir in vanilla. Store in a covered container in the refrigerator.

Yield: About 3 cups. Keeps for about 2 months in the refrigerator.

Melon "Milk"

This refreshing beverage is delicious made with either cantaloupe or honeydew, depending on whether you want your "milk" to be pale orange or green! For a thicker version, blend in some frozen chunks of melon.

> 1 ripe cantaloupe or ½ of a honeydew, halved and seeded

1. Use a spoon to scoop the fruit into your food processor or blender. Blend until smooth and creamy. Serve immediately.

Yield: 1 to 2 servings.

Variation: *Remove seeds from 2 cups watermelon chunks. Blend until smooth.*

Rice Milk

A blender is much better than a food processor for this recipe.

> 2 cups long grain rice (basmati or texmati rice is less starchy)
> 4 cups boiling water (for soaking the rice)
> 5 to 6 cups additional fresh water at room temperature
> 1 to 2 tbsp honey
> 1 tsp vanilla extract

1. Place rice in a strainer and rinse thoroughly under cold running water. Transfer rice to a large bowl. Add boiling water and let soak for 1 to 2 hours, or even overnight. Drain, discarding the water.
2. In a blender, blend 1 cup of the drained rice with 2 ½ cups of fresh water on high speed, about 2 to 3 minutes, until liquefied. Pour into a large bowl. Repeat with remaining rice and 2 ½ cups additional fresh water.

3.   Strain rice milk through a strainer lined with cheesecloth. To speed up the process, press mixture with the back of a spoon. If desired, an additional cup of water can be poured over the rice pulp to produce more milk. Discard rice pulp.

4.   Let rice milk sit for a few minutes. Any sediment will settle to the bottom of the bowl and can be discarded. Flavor rice milk with honey and vanilla. Store in a covered jar in the refrigerator. Shake or stir well before using.

Yield: About 5 to 6 cups. This keeps for 4 to 5 days in the refrigerator.

Variations:
- *If desired, add a pinch of non-iodized salt and a few drops of canola oil.*
- *Sometimes homemade rice milk has a chalky taste. If so, just add a ripe banana and purée well.*
- *Brown basmati rice can be substituted for long grain rice; ¼ cup blanched almonds can replace ¼ cup of the rice.*
- *Chocolate Rice Milk: Add a tablespoon of Easy Chocolate Syrup (see recipe, page 55) and mix well. Yummy!*

■ FRUIT DISHES

Fruit dishes for breakfast make sense on a LID. They're high in fiber, vitamins—and flavor! Many of these recipes are listed in the dessert sections (chapter 7). But fruit-based desserts also make fabulous breakfasts. It's undiscovered territory you'll love!

Basic Baked Apples
(See recipe, page 227.)

Blueberry Apple Crisp
(See recipe, page 221.)

Dried Fruit Compote
(See recipe, page 227.)

Easy Apple Crisp
(See recipe, page 223.)

Easy Pear Crisp
(See recipe, page 223.)

Easy Rhubarb Strawberry Crisp
(See recipe, page 224.)

Homemade Applesauce
(See recipe, page 228.)

Jumbleberry Crisp
(See recipe, page 224.)

Microwave Grapefruit
Cut grapefruit in half. Sprinkle each half with 1 tsp white sugar or drizzle with maple syrup. Place in dessert dishes and microwave uncovered on HIGH for 1 to 1 ¼ minutes. Half a grapefruit will take about 45 seconds to heat. Yummy!

Peachy Crumb Crisp
(See recipe, page 225.)

Pecan Apple Crisp
(See recipe, page 226.)

Poached Pears
(See recipe, page 230.)

Stewed Prunes
(See recipe, page 230.)

Stewed Rhubarb
(See recipe, page 231.) Yes you CAN have rhubarb! See Dr. Ain's Introduction.

Strawberry or Raspberry Purée
(See recipe, page 232.) Perfect with Basic Sweet Egg White Omelet, pancakes and crêpes, or over sliced peaches, nectarines, mangoes or fresh berries.

Summertime Fresh Fruit Compote
(See recipe, page 232.)

■ EGG WHITE DISHES

Basic Savory Egg White Omelet

4 to 6 egg whites
non-iodized salt, to taste
pepper, to taste

1. Combine egg whites with seasonings and mix lightly to blend. Prepare in a frying pan, using olive oil or a LID-safe margarine (see chapter 1). Add any of the following ingredients for the most popular egg/omelet mixtures: chopped asparagus, broccoli, red or green peppers, onions, mushrooms, sliced or diced cooked chicken, zucchini, spinach, tomatoes, Italian herbs, SALT-FREE tomato sauce or hot sauce, Low Iodine Ketch-up (see recipe, page 183).

Basic Sweet Egg White Omelet

4 to 6 egg whites
1 tsp white sugar, if desired

1. Combine egg whites with sugar and mix lightly to blend. Prepare in a
    frying pan using non-stick cooking spray, canola or neutral-flavored
    vegetable oil. Serve plain, and add any of the following as toppings:
    cinnamon/sugar, honey, apple butter, apples, berries, bananas, jams or
    jellies, cranberry sauce, Strawberry or Raspberry Purée (see page 232).

Egg Whites, Any Style

4 to 6 egg whites
non-iodized salt and pepper, to taste

1. Combine egg whites with seasonings and mix lightly to blend. Prepare
    the egg whites as you would normally: fried or scrambled, with the excep-
    tion of sunny-side-up or over-easy! Serve plain or on matzo, or with LID-
    safe bread you may have made or purchased.

Hard-Cooked Egg Whites

How egg-citing—hard-cooked eggs! Use these in a sandwich filling, homemade potato salad or anywhere you use hard-boiled eggs. Two egg whites are
the equivalent of 1 egg.

1. Mix 2 egg whites lightly in a 10 oz glass custard cup or small microsafe
    bowl. Cover tightly with microsafe plastic wrap. Do not vent.
2. Microwave on MEDIUM (50%) for 1 to 1 ½ minutes, depending on
    how powerful your microwave oven is. Let stand covered for 1 to 2
    minutes, until completely set.

Yield: 1 serving. Do not freeze.

■ PANCAKES AND CRÊPES

Apple Cinnamon Pancakes

These are delicious and they're good for you, too! They're sure to become a family favorite.

1 large apple, peeled and cored
1 ⅓ cups flour (part whole wheat flour can be used)
3 tbsp white sugar
1 tsp cinnamon
¼ tsp non-iodized salt
1 tsp baking powder
½ tsp baking soda
1 ¼ cups apple juice
2 tbsp canola oil
2 egg whites (or 3 tbsp pasteurized liquid egg whites)

1. Grate apple; set aside. Combine dry ingredients in a large mixing bowl or food processor and mix until combined. Add apple juice, oil and egg whites. Whisk together (or process for 8 to 10 seconds), just until smooth and blended. Do not overmix. Stir in grated apple.
2. Drop mixture from a large spoon onto a hot, lightly greased griddle or skillet to form pancakes. Cook on medium heat until bubbles appear on the top side, about 2 to 3 minutes. Turn pancakes over carefully with a spatula and brown on the other side. Repeat with remaining batter, greasing pan between batches.

Yield: About 20 three-inch pancakes. Serve with maple syrup or honey. Freezes and/or reheats well. Also see Chef's Tips (page 65).

Blueberry Pancakes

Follow recipe for Easy Pancakes (see page 64), but stir ½ cup fresh or frozen blueberries into batter.

Broccoli Pancakes
(See recipe, page 96.)

Carrots-for-Breakfast Pancakes
Different and delicious!

> 6 medium carrots, peeled
> 1 onion
> 6 egg whites
> 1 tbsp canola oil
> ¾ tsp non-iodized salt
> dash of pepper
> ½ cup flour
> ½ tsp baking powder
> additional oil for frying

1. Cut carrots to fit feed tube of food processor and grate, using firm pressure. Measure 2 cups. Insert Steel Blade in processor bowl. Process onion until fine, about 6 to 8 seconds. Add remaining ingredients except oil for frying. Process until blended, about 15 seconds.
2. Heat oil to ⅛ inch depth in a large skillet. Drop carrot mixture from a large spoon into hot oil, and flatten patties with the back of the spoon. Fry on medium heat about 2 to 3 minutes on each side, until golden brown. Drain well on paper toweling.

Yield: 16 to 18 patties. Freezes well. (To reheat, place patties on a foil-lined cookie sheet and bake uncovered at 450°F for 8 to 10 minutes.)

Note: *Miniatures make an excellent hors d'oeuvre for a cocktail party. Yield in this case is about five dozen.*

Crêpes

These tender crêpes are extremely versatile. This recipe makes a small batch, but it can be doubled easily.

> 2 egg whites (or 3 tbsp pasteurized liquid egg whites)
> ⅓ cup all-purpose flour
> ⅓ cup water
> 1 tbsp canola oil
> pinch of non-iodized salt
> ½ tsp white sugar (for sweet crêpes)

1. In a food processor fitted with the Steel Blade, process egg whites for 4 or 5 seconds. Add remaining ingredients and process 8 to 10 seconds, just until blended. (If you don't have a processor, use a whisk to blend ingredients together.) Let batter stand for 10 to 15 minutes. This helps create a tender crêpe.

2. Brush a 5 or 6 inch crepe pan or skillet lightly with oil. Heat pan on medium-high heat for 2 minutes. Sprinkle with a few drops of water. If water sizzles and bounces off, the pan is hot enough. Quickly pour about 2 tbsp batter into pan. Tilt pan in all directions to coat bottom evenly with batter. Immediately pour any excess batter back into bowl.

3. Cook over medium-high heat about 30 seconds, just until crêpe looks dry. Flip with a spatula and cook briefly on the second side. Fill as desired, roll up and serve.

Yield: 5 or 6 crêpes, depending on size. Freezes and/or reheats well.

Serving Suggestions:

- *For breakfast or brunch, spread crêpes with jam or preserves. Roll up and serve.*
- *For dessert, top them with stewed fruit or berries.*
- *For a main dish, fill crêpes with cooked chicken and/or sautéed vegetables (e.g., mushrooms, onions, broccoli, asparagus). If desired, top with Quick and Easy Tomato Sauce (see page 192). Let your imagination be your guide!*
- *Crêpes reheat very quickly in the microwave, about 10 to 12 seconds each. You can also place filled crêpes seam-side down in a sprayed baking dish and place them in a 350°F oven for a few minutes, until heated through.*

Easy Pancakes

These are very easy to mix up and make an excellent breakfast or brunch dish.

> 1 ¼ cups all-purpose flour (part whole wheat flour can be used)
> 1 tbsp white sugar
> ½ tsp non-iodized salt
> 1 tsp baking powder
> ½ tsp baking soda
> 1 ¼ cups orange juice
> 1 tsp grated orange zest, if desired
> 2 tbsp canola oil
> 2 egg whites (or 3 tbsp pasteurized liquid egg whites)

1. Combine dry ingredients in a large mixing bowl or food processor and mix until combined. Add orange juice, zest, oil and egg whites. Whisk together (or process for 8 to 10 seconds), just until smooth and blended. Do not overmix.

2. Drop mixture from a large spoon onto a hot, lightly greased griddle or
   skillet to form pancakes. Cook on medium heat until bubbles appear on
   the top side, about 2 to 3 minutes. Turn pancakes over carefully with a
   spatula and brown on the other side. Repeat with remaining batter,
   greasing pan between batches.

Yield: About 18 to 20 three-inch pancakes. Serve with maple syrup, honey or
Easy Chocolate Syrup (see page 55). Freezes and/or reheats well.

Chef's Tips:
- *Flour can vary in moisture content, so if your pancake batter is too thick,
  dilute it with a little water. If batter is too thin, add a little flour.*
- *To test if the griddle or skillet is hot enough, sprinkle with a few drops of
  water. If it sizzles and bounces off, your pan is hot enough. If it evaporates,
  your pan is too hot.*
- *Children get very excited when you write their initials with pancake batter.
  Pour batter into the hot skillet to form the desired letters of the alphabet. (If
  you put the batter into a resealable plastic bag and cut a hole in the bottom
  corner, this makes the task easier.)*
- *For lighter pancakes, beat egg whites to the soft peak stage. Then fold
  into batter.*
- *Pancakes reheat quickly in the microwave. Allow about 15 seconds per
  pancake on HIGH power. If frozen, you don't have to thaw them first; just
  microwave them a few seconds longer.*

Zucchini-for-Breakfast Pancakes

Follow recipe for Carrot-for-Breakfast Pancakes (page 62), but substitute 3
medium unpeeled zucchini for the carrots. After grating, salt lightly and let
stand for 15 minutes. Press out excess moisture. Continue as directed.

■ HOMEMADE BREADS, MUFFINS, AND CAKES

With bread machines and food processors, making your own breads and other baked goods is no big deal. Make in advance, before you start your LID, freeze, and use as needed.

Best Blueberry Orange Muffins
Scrumptious!

    4 egg whites
    1 cup white sugar
    ¼ cup canola oil
    ½ cup orange juice (or concentrate)
    1 ½ cups flour (you can use part whole wheat)
    1 ½ tsp baking powder
    ⅛ tsp non-iodized salt
    1 tsp grated orange rind, optional
    1 tsp vanilla
    2 cups blueberries (fresh or frozen)
    1 tbsp flour
    2 tbsp white sugar

1. Preheat oven to 375ºF. Beat egg whites, sugar, and oil until well blended, about 2 minutes. Add juice and mix well. Add flour, baking powder, salt, orange rind, and vanilla. Mix just until flour disappears. In a small bowl, combine blueberries with 1 tbsp flour and 2 tbsp white sugar. Gently stir blueberry mixture into batter.
2. Line muffin pan with paper liners. Fill ¾ full with batter. Bake at 375ºF for 22 to 25 minutes, until golden brown.

Yield: 12 muffins. These freeze beautifully, if they don't disappear in a flash!

Cinnamon Nut Topping

Combine ¼ cup white sugar, ¼ cup finely chopped unsalted nuts and ½ tsp cinnamon. Sprinkle on unbaked muffins. This is also delicious sprinkled on hot oatmeal (see page 48) or your favorite cereal.

Cranberry Bread (Bread Machine Method)

This recipe is courtesy of my friend, Maurice Borts, an expert bread machine baker who enjoys creating unusual bread. This is addictive!

> 1 cup water (room temperature)
> 2 tbsp canola oil
> 2 tbsp honey or white sugar
> ¾ tsp non-iodized salt
> ½ cup rolled oats
> ½ cup whole wheat flour
> 2 cups bread flour
> 1 ½ tsp bread machine yeast
> ½ to ¾ cup dried cranberries (to taste)

1. Place all the ingredients (except cranberries) in baking pan of the bread machine in the order given. Select the whole grain cycle or basic bread cycle. Add cranberries 5 minutes before the end of the kneading cycle (most machines beep to let you know when to add additional ingredients).
2. Using oven mitts, remove bread immediately after the bake cycle is finished to prevent crust from getting soggy. Cool bread on a rack. Fill pan immediately with lukewarm water and let soak for easier cleanup.

Yield: 1 loaf (12 or fewer servings). Bread freezes well.

Note About Bread Machine Breads:

Because breads made in a bread machine come in various shapes, it's difficult to determine how many slices a loaf yields. Most machines make bread in the shape of a tall, square column with a rounded top. Some machines make bread that more closely resembles the traditional rectangular loaf.

Dill Onion Bread (Bread Machine Method)

Dill-icious!

    1 cup water (at room temperature)
    3 egg whites
    3 tbsp canola oil
    3 ¼ cups all-purpose flour
    1 ½ tsp dried dill
    1 ½ tsp non-iodized salt
    2 tbsp white sugar
    2 tsp bread machine yeast
    ½ cup chopped onions

1. Place all the ingredients (except chopped onions) in baking pan of the bread machine in the order given. Yeast should not touch salt or liquids. Select the basic bread cycle. Add onions 5 minutes before the end of the kneading cycle (most machines beep to let you know when to add additional ingredients).
2. Using oven mitts, remove bread immediately after the bake cycle is finished to prevent crust from getting soggy. Remove bread from pan; cool on a rack. Fill pan with lukewarm water and soak for easier cleanup.

Yield: 1 loaf (12 or less servings). Bread freezes well. See note about bread machine, above.

Homemade Whole Wheat Bread
Wholesome and hearty.

1 tsp white sugar

½ cup warm water (about 110°F)

1 package yeast (regular or quick-rise; about 1 tbsp)

1 ⅓ cups all-purpose flour

1 ½ cups whole wheat flour (about)

¼ cup wheat germ, optional

1 ½ tbsp white sugar or honey

1 tbsp non-iodized salt

1 tbsp canola oil

¾ cup lukewarm water

1. Dissolve sugar in ½ cup warm water. Sprinkle yeast over water and let stand 8 to 10 minutes. Stir to dissolve. Measure flours into processor bowl. Add wheat germ, sugar, salt, and oil. Process 10 seconds. Add dissolved yeast; process 10 seconds more. Add ¾ cup lukewarm water slowly through feed tube while machine is running. Process until dough gathers around the blades in a mass. Process 45 seconds longer. Dough should be slightly sticky. If machine slows down, add 3 or 4 tbsp more flour.

2. Turn dough out onto a lightly floured surface. Knead for 2 minutes, until smooth and elastic. Shape into a ball and place in a large lightly greased bowl. Cover bowl with plastic wrap and let dough rise in a warm place until doubled, about 1 ½ to 2 hours. Punch down.

3. Roll or pat dough on a lightly floured board into a 9 inch by 12 inch rectangle. Roll up jelly roll-style from the short side. Seal ends by pressing down with the edge of your hand. Place seam-side down in a sprayed 9 inch by 5 inch loaf pan or on a sprayed baking sheet. Cover with a towel and let rise until it has doubled in size, about 1 hour. Bake in a preheated 425°F oven for 25 to 30 minutes. Remove from pan; let cool.

Yield: 1 loaf (16 slices). Freezes well.

Variations:
- **Homemade White Bread:** *Substitute all-purpose flour for whole wheat flour.*
- **Dinner Rolls:** *In Step 3, shape dough into 12 balls. Place on a sprayed or non-stick cookie sheet, cover and let rise until doubled in size. Bake at 375ºF for 20 minutes, or until golden.*
- **Herb Bread:** *In Step 1, add ½ tsp each of dried basil, dill, thyme, oregano, and/or rosemary to flour. Add remaining ingredients; mix, shape, and bake as directed.*
- **Cinnamon Buns:** *In Step 3, sprinkle dough with ½ cup cinnamon-sugar and ½ cup raisins. Roll up and slice in 1 inch pieces. Place in a sprayed 10 inch spring form pan, with buns barely touching. Brush with melted apricot jam. Cover and let rise until doubled in size. Bake at 375ºF for 30 minutes. When baked, the rolls will be joined together and can be pulled apart easily.*

LID-Safe Baking Dough
This dough is like your basic black dress or suit; it will take you anywhere!

1 tsp white sugar
½ cup warm water (105 to 115ºF)
1 package yeast (about 1 tbsp)
3 cups flour (approximately)
1 tsp non-iodized salt
1 to 3 tbsp white sugar (see tips on following page)
2 to 4 tbsp oil (see tips on following page)
¾ cup lukewarm water

1. Dissolve 1 tsp sugar in ½ cup warm water; mix well. Sprinkle yeast over and let stand for 8 to 10 minutes, until foamy. Stir to dissolve.
2. Steel Blade: Place flour, yeast mixture, salt, sugar and oil in processor bowl. Process 6 to 8 seconds. Add water through the feed tube while the

machine is running. Process until dough gathers together and forms a mass around the blades. (It's better if dough is stickier rather than drier.) Let machine knead dough for 30 to 45 seconds. If machine slows down, add 2 to 4 tbsp flour through the feed tube.

3.   Turn out dough onto a lightly oiled counter. Knead for 1 to 2 minutes until smooth and elastic. Place in a large, lightly greased bowl. Cover with plastic wrap and let rise until it doubles in bulk, about 1 to 2 hours. Punch down. If desired, rise dough a second time. (I usually don't bother.)

4.   Shape dough into bread, rolls, cinnamon buns, or whatever you like. Place on a greased baking pan. Cover with a towel. Cover with plastic wrap and let rise until double in bulk, about 1 hour at room temperature. (For pizza, dough doesn't have to double; you'll have enough dough to make two 12-inch pizzas.) Bake as directed.

Tips and Variations:

- *Use maximum amounts of white sugar and oil if dough will be used for cinnamon buns or sweet breads. Use minimum amounts to make bread, dinner rolls, or pizza.*
- *For cinnamon buns or sweet breads, use maximum amounts of white sugar and oil; add 2 to 3 egg whites along with the ¾ cup lukewarm water.*
- *For breads, dinner rolls or pizza, use minimum amounts of sugar and oil. Do not add any egg whites.*
- *For a more nutritious dough, whole wheat flour can replace half of the all-purpose flour. If desired, add up to ¼ cup wheat germ and/or ground flaxseed.*
- *Baking times: Bread takes 25 to 30 minutes at 400ºF. Rolls take about 18 to 20 minutes. Cinnamon buns take about 20 to 30 minutes at 375ºF, depending on size. When done, breads, rolls, or buns should be golden brown and sound hollow when lightly tapped.*

Magical Carrot Muffins

My friend Roz Brown shared her recipe for these versatile muffins. They'll disappear like magic!

1 ½ cups whole wheat flour (all-purpose flour can replace part of the flour)
⅛ tsp non-iodized salt
1 ½ tsp baking soda
1 tsp cinnamon
¾ cup wheat bran
¾ cup oat bran
1 cup grated carrots (about 3 medium)
4 egg whites
¼ cup canola oil
1 ½ cups orange juice
2 tbsp lemon juice
⅔ cup maple syrup or honey
¾ cup raisins or cut-up prunes

1.	Preheat oven to 375ºF. Combine dry ingredients and blend well. Add carrots, egg whites, and oil. Mix until blended. Add orange juice, lemon juice, maple syrup, or honey and raisins (or prunes). Mix just until blended. Line muffin cups with paper liners. Fill ¾ full with batter. Bake at 375ºF for 20 to 25 minutes, until golden brown.

Yield: 18 muffins. These freeze well.

No-Knead Cinnamon Coffee Cake (Babka)

This is a reduced fat version of my mother's easy-to-prepare yeast coffee cake. No need to knead or punch down the dough. The only rising that's necessary is done right in the baking pan. What could be easier?

1 tsp white sugar

¼ cup warm water (110ºF)

1 package active dry yeast (about 1 tbsp)

3 cups all-purpose flour

½ cup white sugar

½ tsp non-iodized salt

4 egg whites

1 cup lukewarm water

4 tbsp canola oil

¾ cup raisins or chopped dried apricots, rinsed and drained

2 tsp cinnamon

1 tbsp unsweetened pure cocoa powder (LID-safe)

⅓ cup additional white sugar

1. Dissolve sugar in ¼ cup warm water. Add yeast and let stand until foamy, about 8 to 10 minutes. Stir to dissolve. Place flour, sugar, and salt in processor bowl fitted with the Steel Blade. While machine is running, add egg whites, dissolved yeast mixture, lukewarm water and oil through the feed tube. Process for 1 ½ minutes, stopping machine once or twice to scrape down the sides of the bowl. Batter will be very sticky and will drop down in a sheet from a rubber spatula. Add raisins or apricots and process 10 seconds longer.

2. Spray a 10 inch Bundt or springform pan with non-stick spray. Spread half of batter in pan. Combine cinnamon, cocoa, and white sugar; mix well. Sprinkle half over batter. Drop remaining batter by spoonfuls to cover the cinnamon mixture. Sprinkle with remaining cinnamon mixture. Cover with a towel and let rise about 2 hours, until doubled in size. Dough should reach the top of the pan.

3. Preheat oven to 350ºF. Bake for 45 to 50 minutes, until golden. Let cool for 20 minutes, then remove from pan. Cool completely.

Yield: 16 servings. Freezes well.

Oat Bran Muffins

This healthy muffin is high in fiber and pectin, as well as low in cholesterol. Oat bran is an excellent way to help reduce cholesterol levels.

Cinnamon Nut Topping (optional; see page 67)
2 ¼ cups oat bran cereal
1 ½ tsp cinnamon
1 tbsp baking powder
1 apple, peeled and cored (or 2 medium carrots)
¼ cup canola oil
¼ cup honey
1 ¼ cups apple juice
2 egg whites
½ cup raisins, dried cranberries, or unsalted chopped nuts

1. Prepare topping; set aside. Process oat bran on the Steel Blade of the food processor for 1 minute (this makes a muffin with a finer texture). Blend in cinnamon and baking powder. Empty into a mixing bowl. Process apple or carrots until finely minced. Add to oat bran mixture. Add remaining ingredients except topping. Mix just until blended. Do not overmix or muffins will be tough.
2. Fill greased or paper-lined muffin tins ¾ full. Sprinkle with topping, if desired.
3. Bake in a preheated 400°F oven for 18 to 20 minutes. When done, a toothpick will come out dry.

Yield: 10 to 12 medium muffins. These freeze well.

■ DESSERTS FOR BREAKFAST, AGAIN

The following cakes are listed in the dessert section, but are also great for breakfast. Mix with a raw fruit, and you're set!

18-Carrot Cake (or Muffins)
(See recipe, page 205.)

Banana Cake
(See recipe, page 207.)

Lemon Loaf
(See recipe, page 210.)

Lemon Poppy Seed Cake
(See recipe, page 210.)

Whole Wheat Pitas
(See recipe, page 248.)

Yummy Apple Cake
(See recipe, page 211.)

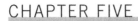

CHAPTER FIVE

LUNCHES
THE EASIEST MEALS

WHAT'S INSIDE

■ SOUPS

Avocado Cucumber Soup

Low-calorie cucumber balances out the high-calorie avocado!

2 medium onions, chopped
2 tbsp canola or vegetable oil
2 cucumbers, peeled, seeded, and diced
2 tbsp minced parsley
2 cloves garlic, minced
4 cups SALT-FREE chicken broth or broth from Free Chicken Soup
(for recipe, see page 83)
1 tsp non-iodized salt
freshly ground pepper to taste
¼ tsp dried basil
¼ tsp dried oregano
dash of cayenne (to taste)
3 ripe avocados, peeled and pitted

1. Combine onions and oil in a 2-quart microsafe bowl or casserole.
    Microwave uncovered on HIGH for 3 to 4 minutes, stirring at half time.
    Add cucumbers, parsley, and garlic. Microwave covered on HIGH for 5
    minutes, until cucumbers are fairly soft.
2. Add chicken broth along with seasonings. Cover and microwave on
    HIGH for 15 minutes.
3. Purée avocado on the Steel Blade of the food processor until smooth.
    Strain hot cucumber mixture, reserving liquid. Add cucumber mixture
    to processor and process until smooth. Add to reserved liquid and blend
    well. Adjust seasonings to taste.

Yield: 6 servings. Delicious hot or cold.

Beef Barley Soup

6 or 8 strips short ribs (flanken)
3 quarts cold water (12 cups)
1 tbsp non-iodized salt
2 onions, quartered
3 stalks celery, cut in 2 inch chunks
½ turnip, cut in 1 inch chunks
3 carrots, scraped and cut in 1 inch chunks
1 ¼ cups barley
¼ tsp pepper

1. Place short ribs in a large soup pot. Add cold water and salt. Bring to a boil and skim well.
2. Steel Blade: Process onions and celery in a food processor until finely minced, about 6 to 8 seconds. Add to soup. Repeat with turnip and carrots. Add remaining ingredients to soup. Cover and simmer slowly for 3 hours. Taste to correct seasonings.

Yield: 10 to 12 hearty servings. May be frozen. Thin soup with a little water if necessary when reheating.

Cabbage Soup with Meatballs

You can "grate" the cabbage quickly in a food processor with the slicing blade, using very light pressure.

2 ½ quarts boiling water (10 cups)
28 oz can SALT-FREE tomatoes
5 ½ oz can SALT-FREE tomato paste
8 oz can SALT-FREE tomato sauce
1 lb lean ground beef
¾ tsp non-iodized salt

freshly ground pepper
2 egg whites
2 tbsp matzo meal or rolled oats
¼ tsp garlic powder or 1 clove garlic, minced
1 onion, thinly sliced or grated
½ head cabbage, cored and thinly sliced
½ cup white sugar (or to taste)
2 tbsp lemon juice
non-iodized salt and ground pepper, to taste
½ cup rice, if desired

1. Combine water, canned tomatoes, tomato paste, and tomato sauce in a large soup pot and bring to a boil.
2. In a large mixing bowl, combine ground beef, salt, pepper, egg whites, matzo meal or rolled oats, and garlic powder. Shape into tiny meatballs and add to soup pot.
3. Add onion and cabbage to soup along with remaining ingredients except rice. Cover and simmer for about 2 ½ hours. Add rice and simmer 25 minutes longer. Adjust seasonings to taste.

Yield: 12 to 16 hearty servings. If soup is too thick, a little water may be added. May be frozen.

Tip: *If desired, make double the amount of meatballs, and serve this as a meal-in-a-bowl.*

Chicken Spaghetti Soup

4 single chicken breasts with bone (skin removed)
6 cups cold water
1 tbsp non-iodized salt
3 to 4 cloves garlic

1 large onion, cut in chunks
2 carrots, cut in chunks
2 stalks celery, cut in chunks
½ cup green split peas
¼ cup barley, rinsed and drained
5 ½ oz can SALT-FREE tomato paste
28 oz can SALT-FREE tomatoes
2 bay leaves
freshly ground pepper
1 tsp Italian seasoning (or ½ tsp each dried basil and oregano)
¼ tsp each dried rosemary and thyme
1 cup fresh green beans, if desired
2 additional carrots
1 cup SALT-FREE canned kidney beans, well-drained
14 oz can SALT-FREE green peas
1 ½ to 2 cups spaghetti, broken into pieces

1. Place chicken in cold salted (using non-iodized salt)
    water in a large soup pot. Bring to a boil. Skim.
2. Steel Blade: Drop garlic through feed tube of food processor while
    machine is running. Process until minced. Add onion, carrots, and celery
    and process until fine. Add to soup. Add split peas, barley, tomato paste,
    and canned tomatoes. Season, cover and simmer for 2 hours,
    stirring occasionally.
3. Slicer: Cut green beans to fit crosswise in feed tube. Slice, using firm
    pressure. Slice additional carrots, using firm pressure. Add all remaining
    ingredients to soup. Simmer about 25 minutes longer, stirring occasion-
    ally. Adjust seasonings.

Yield: 12 hearty servings. May be frozen.

Chicken, Lima Bean and Barley Soup
(See recipe, page 124.)

Chilled Beet Soup

2 ½ lb beets, peeled
1 onion
2 quarts cold water (8 cups)
19 oz can SALT-FREE tomato juice or 2 ½ cups fresh tomato juice (5 to 6 tomatoes, processed until liquefied)
2 tbsp lemon juice
1 cup white sugar
2 tsp non-iodized salt
a few sprigs fresh dill or parsley

1. Grater: Cut beets to fit feed tube of food processor. Grate, using fairly firm pressure. (A slight bouncing motion with the pusher is best.) Grate onion. Combine beets and onion in a large saucepan with water. Bring to a boil, reduce heat to a simmer and add remaining ingredients.
2. Simmer for 1 hour partially covered. Taste to adjust seasoning. Refrigerate. Serve chilled with fresh parsley or dill. If desired, add a light drizzle of olive oil on top. Will keep for 2 to 3 weeks in the refrigerator in a tightly closed container.

Yield: 8 servings. Freezes well.

Country Vegetable Soup
(See recipe, page 125.)

Free Chicken Soup

Buy chicken breasts with skin and bones. Use the boneless breasts in your favorite recipes. Save the skin and bones to make this soup! Be sure to make it at least a day in advance so you can discard the congealed fat.

skin and bones from 8 whole raw chicken breasts
8 cups cold water
3 to 4 tsp non-iodized salt (to taste)
¼ tsp pepper
4 to 6 carrots, scraped and trimmed
3 stalks celery
1 large onion
6 sprigs dill

1. Combine skin, bones and cold water in a large pot. Add salt and bring to a boil. Skim. Add remaining ingredients, cover, and simmer for about 2 hours. Strain and refrigerate overnight. Discard skin and bones.
2. Remove the fat that congeals on top and discard. Reheat soup and serve with LID Soup Dumplings (see recipe, page 131), LID-safe noodles or rice.

Yield: 6 to 8 servings. Freezes well.

Garden Vegetable Soup
(See recipe, page 127.)

Homemade Beef or Veal Broth
(See recipe, page 128.)

Jewish Soup Dumplings (matzo balls)
(See recipe, page 130.)

LID Soup Dumplings
(See recipe, page 131.)

Luscious Lentil Soup
(See recipe, page 131.)

Mushroom Barley Soup
Follow recipe for Vegetable Barley Soup (see page 87), but add 2 cups sliced mushrooms along with the barley. Canned tomatoes can be omitted, but increase water to 10 cups.

Potato Mushroom Soup
An old European recipe that has been adapted for the food processor.

    2 onions, quartered
    2 tbsp olive oil
    4 or 5 medium potatoes, pared
    1 pint mushrooms (about 2 ½ cups)
    5 cups boiling water
    1 tsp non-iodized salt
    freshly ground pepper

1. Steel Blade: Process onions with 3 or 4 quick on/off turns, until coarsely chopped. Heat oil in a heavy 3-quart saucepan. Add onions and sauté for 5 minutes on medium heat, until golden.
2. Slicer: Cut potatoes to fit feed tube. Slice, using medium pressure. Slice mushrooms, using medium pressure. Add all ingredients to saucepan, cover and simmer for 20 to 25 minutes, until tender, stirring occasionally.

Yield: 4 to 6 servings. May be frozen.

Purée of Red Pepper Soup

Arlene Ward, a dynamic cooking teacher from New York, shared her recipe with me over dinner at a convention of the International Association of Cooking Professionals in St. Louis. The other teachers at the table added bits and pieces, and I converted the recipe for the microwave.

    3 tbsp olive oil
    2 cloves garlic, minced
    2 leeks (white part), sliced
    2 lb red peppers, halved, seeded and cut in chunks
    3 cups SALT-FREE chicken broth or broth from Free Chicken Soup
    (for recipe, see page 83)
    non-iodized salt and ground pepper, to taste
    ½ tsp sugar
    dash of cayenne (or to taste)

1. Pour olive oil into a 2 quart microsafe bowl or casserole. Stir in garlic, leeks and peppers. Microwave uncovered on HIGH for 6 to 7 minutes, until tender-crisp, stirring at half time.
2. Add remaining ingredients. Microwave covered on HIGH for 15 minutes, until peppers are tender. Purée through a food mill or strainer to remove skins from peppers. Adjust seasonings to taste.

Yield: 4 servings. May be frozen.

Tip: *For special company, make one batch of soup with red peppers and another with yellow peppers. Cut a strip of heavy-duty foil the diameter of your soup bowl, folding it so it's strong enough to stand upright on its own. Place in soup bowl. Pour red soup on one side of the foil and yellow soup on the other side. Remove the foil before serving, of course!*

Quick Gazpacho
(Chilled Tomato-Based Soup)

This refreshing soup is made very quickly in a food processor!

1 large cucumber, peeled
1 green pepper, seeded
1 onion
6 tomatoes, peeled and cored
4 cloves garlic
juice of ½ lemon
¼ cup olive or canola oil
½ tsp each chili powder and basil
1 tbsp non-iodized salt
19 oz can SALT-FREE tomato juice or 2 ½ cups fresh tomato juice
(6 to 8 tomatoes, processed until liquefied)

1. Cut cucumber, green pepper, onion, and tomatoes into large chunks.
2. Steel Blade: Process cucumber with 4 or 5 on/off turns, until finely chopped. Transfer to a large bowl. Repeat with green pepper, then onion, then tomatoes, adding each in turn to the mixing bowl.
3. Drop garlic through feed tube while machine is running. Process until minced. Add lemon juice, oil, chili powder, basil, salt, and half of the tomato juice. Process until smooth. Add to chopped vegetables along with remaining tomato juice. Adjust seasonings to taste.
4. Chill for several hours in order to blend flavors. This will keep very well in the refrigerator in a tightly closed jar. Serve with additional chopped vegetables, if desired.

Yield: 6 servings.

The Best Chicken Soup

(See recipe, page 133.)

Vegetable Barley Soup

Use your food processor to make quick work of preparing the vegetables.

2 lb flanken (short ribs), stewing beef, or veal, well-trimmed
8 cups water
2 onions, chopped
1 potato or sweet potato, peeled and chopped
3 carrots, sliced
3 stalks celery, sliced
28 oz can SALT-FREE tomatoes or 6 fresh tomatoes, puréed
1 tbsp non-iodized salt
½ tsp pepper
½ tsp thyme
½ cup pearl barley, rinsed and drained
1 cup split peas, rinsed and drained (optional)
¼ cup fresh parsley or dill, minced (to garnish)

1. If using short ribs, cut in pieces. If using stewing meat, cut in 1-inch pieces. Place meat and water in a large soup pot and bring to a boil. Skim well; reduce heat to low.
2. Add remaining ingredients except parsley or dill to soup pot; break up tomatoes with a spoon. Cover partially and simmer for 3 hours, until meat and barley are tender. Stir occasionally during cooking. If soup is too thick, add a little water. Adjust seasonings to taste. Flavor is even better the next day. Garnish with parsley or dill at serving time.

Yield: 10 to 12 servings. Freezes well.

Vegetable Broth ("Almost Chicken Soup")

(See recipe, page 134.)

Vegetarian "Chicken" Broth
(See recipe, page 134.)

■ SALADS

Balsamic Salad Splash
An almost fat-free dressing. Perfect over salad greens.

> ¼ cup balsamic vinegar
> ¼ cup water
> ¼ cup honey
> ¼ tsp garlic powder
> dash of cayenne (to taste)
> 2 tsp olive or canola oil

1. Combine all ingredients in a jar; shake well. Refrigerate until needed. Shake well before serving.

Yield: about ¾ cup. Dressing can be stored in the refrigerator for up to a month.

Best Bean Salad
This is a great do-ahead recipe. Even though it may seem long, it's very easy to prepare. Try it, you'll love it!

> 2 cups fresh green beans
> 2 cups fresh wax beans
> ½ cup water
> 10 oz package frozen, SALT-FREE baby lima beans
> 19 oz can SALT-FREE chickpeas, drained (or 2 cups cooked chickpeas)
> ½ cup canned SALT-FREE red kidney beans (or ½ cup cooked kidney beans)
> ½ of a Spanish or Vidalia onion, chopped

½ of a red pepper, seeded and chopped
½ of a green pepper, seeded and chopped
2 or 3 cloves garlic, crushed

Dressing:
1 cup red wine vinegar
½ cup white sugar
½ cup canola oil
1 tsp dry mustard
1 tsp non-iodized salt
freshly ground pepper

1. Wash and trim green beans and wax beans. Cut in 1-inch pieces. Combine with water in a 2-quart round microsafe casserole. Cover and microwave on HIGH for 5 to 7 minutes, stirring halfway through cooking. Beans should be tender-crisp. Let stand covered for 2 to 3 minutes. Rinse well with cold water to stop cooking process. Drain well. (Beans can also be steamed for 5 to 7 minutes.)
2. Pierce top of package of lima beans in several places with a sharp knife. Place on a microsafe plate. Microwave on HIGH for 5 to 7 minutes, shaking in package halfway through cooking to mix lima beans. Let stand covered for 2 minutes. Remove from package and rinse with cold water to stop cooking process. Drain well.
3. Combine all ingredients except dressing in a large bowl.
4. Mix well.
5. Combine all ingredients for dressing in an 8-cup Pyrex measure. Microwave uncovered on HIGH for 3 minutes, stirring at half time, until steaming hot. Pour hot dressing over vegetables and mix well. Refrigerate.

Yield: 12 servings. Keeps about a week to 10 days in the refrigerator.

Note: *A 10 oz package of SALT-FREE frozen green beans and a 10 oz package of*

SALT-FREE frozen wax beans can be used instead of fresh beans in Step 1. Pierce top of each package. Stack one on top of the other in a microsafe dish. Microwave on HIGH for 10 to 12 minutes, switching the packages around halfway through cooking. Let stand for 3 minutes. Rinse under cold water to stop the cooking. Drain well; continue as directed in Step 2.

Best Cole Slaw
(See recipe, page 135.)

Israeli Salad
This scrumptious chopped vegetable salad is always a favorite at a buffet. Recipe can be halved, if desired.

> 1 head of Romaine or iceberg lettuce
> 4 green onions
> 1 medium onion
> 2 green peppers
> 1 red pepper
> 1 English cucumber, peeled
> 8 firm, ripe tomatoes (preferably Israeli or Italian plum/Roma)
> 4 tbsp olive oil (preferably extra-virgin)
> 4 tbsp fresh lemon juice
> non-iodized salt and ground pepper, to taste

1. Wash and dry vegetables well. Dice them neatly into ½-inch pieces and combine in a large bowl. Sprinkle with olive oil and lemon juice. Add seasonings; mix again. Adjust seasonings to taste.

Yield: 8 servings. Salad tastes best eaten the same day it's made, but leftovers will keep for a day in the refrigerator. Drain off excess liquid in the bottom of the bowl before serving.

Mediterranean Vegetable Salad: *Add ½ cup sliced radishes and ½ cup chopped fresh parsley or coriander/cilantro. This is also delicious with finely chopped fresh mint.*

Italiano Dressing

> 1 clove garlic
> 1 cup canola or olive oil
> ¼ cup red wine vinegar
> 1 tbsp lemon juice
> 1 ¼ tsp non-iodized salt
> ¼ tsp freshly ground pepper
> ½ tsp dry mustard
> ¼ tsp dried oregano
> ¼ tsp white sugar
> pinch of dried thyme
> pinch of dried dill weed (or 1 tbsp fresh dill)

1. Steel Blade: Discard garlic peel. Drop garlic through feed tube while machine is running. Process until minced. Scrape down sides of bowl, add remaining ingredients and process until blended, about 5 seconds.

Yield: About 1 ¼ cups dressing. Store in a tightly closed jar in the refrigerator. Keeps about 1 month. Shake before using. Do not freeze.

Marinated Bean Salad

> 1 large Spanish or Bermuda onion
> 1 green pepper, halved and seeded
> 1 red pepper, halved and seeded
> 14 oz can SALT-FREE cut green beans, drained
> 14 oz can SALT-FREE cut wax (yellow) beans, drained
> 10 oz can SALT-FREE baby lima beans, drained

½ cup SALT-FREE canned kidney beans, drained
½ cup olive or canola oil
¼ cup vinegar
non-iodized salt and pepper, to taste
1 tsp dry mustard
2 to 3 tbsp white sugar
2 cups raw cauliflower florets

1. Slicer: Cut onion to fit feed tube of food processor. Slice, using light pressure. Slice peppers, using light pressure. Combine all ingredients and toss to mix. Cover, refrigerate for at least 24 hours before serving.

Yield: about 12 servings. Will keep about 10 days in the refrigerator.

Note: *You may substitute cooked fresh beans for canned, if desired.*

QUICK SOAKING OF DRIED BEANS, PEAS AND LENTILS

Yes, you can have all the beans and legumes you like! (See Dr. Ain's Introduction). There's no need to soak legumes overnight when you use this method. Although some cookbooks tell you that lentils and split peas don't require soaking, all legumes will be much easier to digest if they're presoaked before cooking.

1. Rinse beans, peas or lentils under cold running water in a colander, discarding any shriveled or discolored ones. Cover with triple the amount of cold water in a large saucepan.
2. Bring to a boil, cook 2 minutes. Remove from heat, let stand for 1 hour.
3. Discard any beans that are floating. Cut through one bean with a sharp knife. The interior should be the same color and texture throughout. Otherwise, soak a few minutes longer. Drain and rinse well.
4. Cook in fresh water according to your favorite recipe. (If you use the soaking water to cook them, you may suffer from flatulence!)

Orange Balsamic Vinaigrette

Wonderful on mixed salad greens. It also makes a yummy marinade for boneless chicken breasts.

> ¼ cup olive or canola oil
> 6 tbsp orange juice
> ¼ cup balsamic vinegar
> 1 or 2 cloves garlic, crushed
> 2 tbsp minced fresh basil (or ½ tsp dried)
> 1 tbsp white sugar
> non-iodized salt and ground pepper, to taste

1. Combine all ingredients and mix well. Dressing will keep in the refrigerator about 2 weeks.

Yield: About ¾ cup.

Red Cabbage Cole Slaw

(See recipe, page 137.)

Simply Basic Vinaigrette

A light and luscious vinaigrette salad dressing.

> ¼ cup olive or canola oil
> ¼ cup rice, balsamic or red wine vinegar
> ¼ cup orange juice
> ½ tsp dry mustard
> 1 tbsp honey or maple syrup
> ½ tsp dried basil (or 1 tbsp fresh minced)
> 1 clove garlic, crushed
> non-iodized salt and ground pepper, to taste

1.   Combine all ingredients and mix well. Drizzle over your favorite salad greens and toss to mix.

Yield: About ¾ cup dressing. Leftovers can be refrigerated for up to 2 weeks.

Tip: *Use different herbs to provide different flavor boosts. Substitute dill, thyme, oregano or Italian seasonings for the basil. If dressing is refrigerated, olive oil will congeal. Just let the dressing stand at room temperature for a few minutes before serving and the oil will liquefy; shake well.*

Tomato, Onion, and Pepper Salad

3 or 4 firm, ripe tomatoes, cut in eighths
1 cup thinly sliced Spanish, Vidalia or red onion
½ of a red pepper, sliced
½ of a green pepper, sliced
½ of a yellow pepper, sliced
2 tbsp fresh basil, chopped (or 1 tsp dried basil)
2 cloves garlic, crushed
2 tbsp olive oil (preferably extra-virgin)
2 tbsp fresh lemon juice or balsamic vinegar
non-iodized salt and ground pepper, to taste

1.   Combine tomatoes, onions, peppers, basil, and garlic in a large bowl. (Can be prepared a few hours in advance, covered and refrigerated.) Add remaining ingredients and toss gently. Serve immediately.

Yield: 6 servings. Leftovers will keep about a day in the refrigerator.

Unique and Yummy Vegetable Salad

2 cups green beans
2 cups yellow beans
1 small head cauliflower, broken into florets
1 green pepper, halved and seeded
1 red pepper, halved and seeded
2 Spanish onions, quartered
1 stalk celery, cut to fit feed tube
1 can SALT-FREE artichoke hearts, drained (if desired)

Marinade:
2 cloves garlic
1 cup white vinegar
¼ cup canola or olive oil
½ cup white sugar
2 tsp non-iodized salt

1. Cut beans in half and boil for 2 or 3 minutes in boiling water to cover. Drain well.
2. Slicer: Slice cauliflower, using fairly firm pressure. Slice peppers, onions and celery, using medium pressure. Combine all vegetables in large bowl.
3. Steel Blade: Drop garlic through feed tube while machine is running. Process until minced. Add to saucepan along with vinegar, oil, sugar and salt. Bring mixture to a boil. Pour hot marinade over vegetables and mix well. Store in glass jars in the refrigerator. Will keep about 2 weeks.

Yield: 16 to 20 servings

Variation: *Add 1 unpeeled zucchini and 1 bunch broccoli florets, sliced on the Slicer. If you wish, add 1 large carrot. Pack in feed tube crosswise. Slice with firm pressure. Carrots should be parboiled with the beans before adding to the salad.*

■ VEGETABLE AND SIDE DISHES

Apricot Candied Carrots
(See recipe, page 138.)

Asparagus
(See recipe, page 138.)

Basic Polenta (Cornmeal Mush)
(See recipe and serving suggestions, page 46.)

Broccoli Pancakes

> 10 oz package frozen broccoli (or ½ bunch fresh broccoli, cut
> in chunks)
> 1 small onion, halved
> 6 egg whites
> 1 tbsp olive or canola oil
> ½ cup matzo meal
> ¾ tsp non-iodized salt
> dash pepper
> additional oil for frying

1. Cook frozen broccoli according to package directions. (Cook fresh
   broccoli in boiling salted water until tender.) Drain thoroughly.
2. Steel Blade: Process onion until minced. Scrape down sides of bowl. Add
   egg whites, oil, and broccoli; process until finely chopped, about 20
   seconds. Add matzo meal and seasonings and process a few seconds
   longer, until smooth.

3. Heat about 3 to 4 tbsp oil in a large skillet. Drop in vegetable mixture from a tablespoon to make small pancakes. Flatten slightly with the back of the spoon. Brown on both sides. Drain on paper toweling. Add more oil if necessary.

Yield: about 1 ½ dozen small pancakes. May be frozen.

Corn on the Cob
(See recipe, page 141.)

Eggplant Spread #1
(See recipe, page 251.)

Eggplant Spread #2
(See recipe, page 251.)

Garlic Roasted Carrots

1 large onion, sliced
2 lb carrots, cut in 2-inch lengths
2 to 3 cloves garlic, minced
2 to 3 tbsp olive oil
non-iodized salt and freshly ground pepper, to taste

1. Preheat oven to 375°F. Place onions, carrots, and garlic in a large casserole. Drizzle with olive oil and sprinkle with salt and pepper; mix well.
2. Roast uncovered for 45 to 60 minutes, until golden and tender, stirring occasionally. (For best results, make sure carrots are in a single layer.) Serve hot or at room temperature.

Yield: 4 servings. Do not freeze. Reheats well.

Variations:

- *Add a drizzle of balsamic vinegar or fresh lemon juice. You can add your favorite herbs, such as cumin, minced basil, oregano, dill, rosemary, or paprika; sprinkle with Seasoned Salt (see page 243). If adding fresh herbs, add them during the last 5 minutes of roasting.*
- **Garlic Roasted Carrots and Potatoes:** *Use 1 lb carrots. Add 3 potatoes, peeled and sliced, along with ½ cup of water.*

Green Beans Almondine

(See recipe, page 140.)

Grilled Eggplant Roumanian-Style

2 medium eggplants (about 2 ½ lb)
1 tbsp olive or canola oil
3 tbsp lemon juice or balsamic vinegar
2 cloves garlic, crushed
non-iodized salt to taste
pepper to taste
2 tbsp chopped parsley
¼ cup each chopped red and green pepper
¼ cup chopped green onions

1. Preheat broiler or BBQ. Broil eggplants about 4 inches from the heat on a sprayed baking sheet, or grill them on the BBQ, turning them every 5 minutes, until charred and tender. When cool, peel off skin. Gently squeeze out liquid.
2. Combine all ingredients and beat or process in a food processor until smooth and light. Chill to blend flavors. Serve with LID-safe bread or chips (see Snacks chapter). Also delicious served on a bed of salad greens.

Yield: About 4 cups. Keeps about 3 or 4 days in the refrigerator.

Grilled Lyonnaise Potatoes

4 large potatoes, peeled
2 medium onions
2 tbsp olive or canola oil
non-iodized salt and pepper, to taste
paprika, to taste
2 tbsp fresh parsley

1. Cut a large sheet of heavy-duty aluminum foil, or fold regular-strength foil to double thickness. Insert Slicer in processor. Cut potatoes and onions to fit feed tube. Slice, using medium pressure. Arrange potatoes and onions in a layer about half-inch thick in the center of foil. Drizzle with oil and sprinkle with seasonings.
2. Steel Blade: Chop parsley until minced, about 5 seconds. Sprinkle over potatoes and onions. Wrap foil loosely, sealing all ends well.
3. Barbecue Method: Place on grill about 4 inches from hot coals. Cook about 20 to 30 minutes, turning package halfway through cooking.
4. Oven Method: Bake at 450ºF about 20 minutes. Do not turn.

Yield: 4 servings. Do not freeze.

Honey-Glazed Carrots
(See recipe, page 140.)

Pizza Potato Skins
Did you know that most of the nutrients are just under the skin of the potato? This is an excellent way to enjoy them.

4 medium baking potatoes (e.g., Idaho)
¾ cup SALT-FREE tomato sauce or Fresh Tomato Sauce (see recipe, page 189)

¼ cup chopped green or red pepper
¼ cup chopped mushrooms
¼ cup chopped onions
non-iodized salt and pepper, to taste

1. Scrub potatoes thoroughly; pierce in several places with a sharp knife.
    Bake in a conventional oven at 400ºF until tender, about 1 hour, or
    microwave on HIGH about 10 to 12 minutes, turning them over at half
    time. Cool slightly.
2. Cut potatoes in half horizontally. Scoop out cooked potato and reserve
    for another use. Arrange the potato skins cut-side up in a circle on a large
    microsafe platter. Brush each potato skin with 1 or 2 tbsp tomato sauce.
    Sprinkle with chopped green pepper, mushrooms and onions. Season
    with salt and pepper.
3. Microwave uncovered on HIGH for 2 ½ to 3 minutes (or 30 to 45
    seconds per potato skin). Rotate plate ¼ turn halfway through cooking.
    For a crispy skin on the potatoes, bake in a conventional oven at 400ºF
    for 12 to 15 minutes.

Yield: 2 to 4 servings, depending on who's eating. These reheat well.

Roasted Red Peppers
(See recipe, page 259.)

Smoky Eggplant Dip
(See recipe, page 256.)

Tasty Green Beans
(See recipe, page 146.)

Yum-Yum Potato Wedgies

Crusty outside, fluffy inside: The best of both worlds with a combination of microwave and conventional cooking!

4 medium baking potatoes (about 1 ¾ lb)
1 to 2 tbsp canola or olive oil
non-iodized salt
ground pepper, paprika, and garlic powder

1. Do not peel potatoes, but scrub well. Cut each potato lengthwise into 4 wedges. (Or slice potatoes in rounds about ½ inch thick.) Rinse, but do not dry. Rub oil and seasonings on all surfaces. Arrange in a single layer in a lightly greased oblong Pyrex casserole. Preheat conventional oven to 400ºF.
2. While oven is preheating, microwave potatoes uncovered on HIGH for 10 minutes, until crisp-tender, stirring at half time.
3. Transfer potatoes to the conventional oven. Bake uncovered at 400ºF for 15 to 20 minutes, turning occasionally, until brown and crispy.

Yield: 4 servings. Do not freeze.

■ PASTAS AND SAUCES

Cheater's High-Fiber Pasta Sauce

(See recipe, page 186.)

Fast Pasta with Veggies

Use one pot to cook the pasta and the veggies! It doesn't get much easier or faster than this. The recipe can be doubled easily.

8 ounces LID-safe pasta (e.g., penne or rotini)
boiling water (add non-iodized salt)

2 cups SALT-FREE frozen mixed vegetables (e.g., broccoli, cauliflower, green beans, red pepper)
2 to 3 tbsp good quality olive oil
2 to 3 cloves minced garlic
2 tbsp minced fresh basil (or 1 tsp dried basil)
non-iodized salt and pepper, to taste
red pepper flakes, optional

1. Add pasta to a big pot of boiling water to which you've added non-iodized salt. Cook until almost done, 6 to 7 minutes.
2. Add frozen vegetables to the pot. The water will stop boiling as you add the veggies, then quickly return it to a boil. Continue cooking about 3 or 4 minutes longer until pasta is done and veggies are tender, but still brightly colored.
3. Drain well. Toss with olive oil, garlic, and basil. Season with salt, pepper, and red pepper flakes.

Yield: 2 to 3 servings. Reheats well.

Fresh Tomato Sauce
(See recipe, page 189.)

High-Fiber Vegetarian Pasta Sauce
(See recipe, page 190.)

PASTA-BILITIES
- 8 ounces of uncooked pasta will serve 2 to 3 generously. Any leftovers can be eaten for lunch the next day or can be used as a side dish for dinner.
- For variety, use different shapes of LID-safe pasta.

LID-Safe Homemade Pasta

The processor mixes up this delicious and easy pasta in just 30 seconds! It's easily rolled and cut by hand; if it becomes a habit, invest in a pasta machine.

1 ½ cups all-purpose flour
½ tsp non-iodized salt
4 egg whites
1 ½ tbsp water (approximately)
1 tbsp canola oil

1. Steel Blade: Process flour with salt for 3 or 4 seconds. Add egg whites and water and process about 25 to 30 seconds until dough is well kneaded and forms a ball on the blades. Divide in 4 equal pieces. Roll each piece on a floured board into a 10-inch square. Dough should be as thin as possible. Let dry on towels about 20 minutes, turning each piece of dough over after 10 minutes for more even drying. (You may eliminate drying the pasta, if desired.)
2. Roll up each piece of dough jelly-roll style. Cut with a sharp knife into half-inch wide strips (or whatever width you want noodles to be). Unroll and place on a lightly floured towel to dry for 1 to 2 hours. (The kids love to help unroll the dough and lay it out.) If noodles are to be used immediately, it's not necessary to dry them before cooking.
3. Bring 4 quarts of water to a boil. Add 4 tsp salt. Cook noodles for about 3 or 4 minutes, or until al dente (slightly firm, but done). Cooking time will vary, depending on dryness of noodles. Drain immediately.

Yield: 3 to 4 servings, or about ¾ pound noodles. This is the equivalent of a 12 oz package.

Note: *Uncooked noodles may be frozen up to 1 month, or may be stored for 2 to 3 days in the refrigerator in a plastic bag. Recipe may be doubled successfully and processed in one batch.*

TO USE PASTA MACHINE:

- Crank each piece of dough through the widest setting of machine rollers 3 or 4 times, flouring and folding dough in half each time you run it through. Then reset the rollers and run the pasta through subsequent, ever-narrowing openings, until you have a long, thin length of pasta. (If it becomes too long and awkward to handle, just cut the pasta in half.) Flour the dough from time to time to prevent sticking. Spread on towels to dry for 20 minutes, turning each piece of dough over after 10 minutes. (You may eliminate drying the pasta, if desired.)
- Change handle of the machine from roller to cutter position for thin or wide noodles. Roll pasta through desired cutters. Separate noodles and spread on a towel to dry for at least 15 minutes before cooking, or for 1 to 2 hours if storing. Cook as directed.
- For fettucine: Cut into ½-inch strips. Cook 3 to 4 minutes.
- For lasagna noodles: Make pasta but do not let it dry. Cut into rectangles about 4 ½ inches wide and the same length as your baking dish. (This makes lasagna easy to assemble.) Cooking the pasta in advance is not necessary.
- For cannelloni and manicotti: Cut in 5 inch lengths. Cook about 1 minute. Drain well. Lay flat on towels. Fill as desired.

Noodle Bake

Noodle pudding (also known as kugel) made using only egg whites tends to be paler than those made with whole eggs, but still tastes delicious. To add color, add a dash of paprika to the noodle mixture before baking.

Homemade Pasta (See recipe, page 103) or,
12 oz package medium or egg-free broad noodles
¼ cup canola oil
1 large onion, chopped

8 egg whites or 1 cup pasteurized liquid egg whites
non-iodized salt and pepper, to taste

1. Cook noodles according to package or recipe directions. Drain well. Return to saucepan. Heat oil in a 7- by 11-inch Pyrex baking dish at 425ºF.
2. Stir chopped onions into hot oil. Leave in oven about 5 minutes, until onions are lightly browned.
3. Beat egg whites with a whisk until frothy. Combine with noodles and seasonings. Stir into oil/onion mixture. Bake uncovered at 400ºF about 1 hour, until golden.

Yield: 8 to 10 servings. Freezes well.

Variation: *For a lighter texture, add 1 cup SALT-FREE chicken broth to the noodle/egg white mixture in Step 3.*

Noodle Apple Bake

Make Noodle Bake (see page 104), but eliminate onion. Peel and core 3 apples. Insert Grater in processor. Grate apples, using medium pressure. Add grated apples, ⅓ cup white sugar and ½ tsp cinnamon to noodle mixture; mix until combined. Bake as directed. May be frozen.

Noodle Raisin Bake

Make Noodle Bake (above), but eliminate onion. Add ½ cup raisins, ½ cup white sugar and 1 tsp cinnamon to noodle mixture. Bake as directed. Freezes well.

Pasta with Pesto and Tomatoes

This is guaranteed to become a family favorite! This can be doubled easily.

8 ounces LID-safe pasta (e.g., bow ties or fettucine)
boiling water

non-iodized salt, as needed

2 tbsp SALT-FREE tomato paste*

1 tbsp olive oil

3 to 4 tbsp Homemade Pesto (see recipe, page 191)

pepper, to taste

2 tomatoes, coarsely chopped

1.   Cook pasta in a big pot of boiling water to which you've added 1 tbsp non-iodized salt. Cook about 8 to 10 minutes until al dente (slightly firm).

2.   Drain well, reserving about ½ cup of the cooking water.

3.   Combine pasta with tomato paste, olive oil, pesto, and some of the cooking water. Season with salt and pepper. Garnish with chopped tomatoes. Serve immediately.

Yield: 2 to 3 servings. Reheats well, either in the microwave oven, or in a non-stick skillet on the stovetop.

Leftover tomato paste can be frozen. Drop by tablespoon in separate dollops onto a wax-paper lined tray and freeze until solid. Transfer dollops to a freezer bag and store in freezer. Use as needed.

Quick and Easy Tomato Sauce (Vegetarian Spaghetti Sauce)
(See recipe, page 192.)

Un-Can-ny Spaghetti Sauce

3 cloves garlic

2 medium onions, quartered

3 tbsp canola or olive oil

1 green pepper, halved and seeded

1 cup mushrooms, if desired
2 lb lean ground beef
28 oz can SALT FREE tomatoes
2 – 5 ½ oz cans SALT-FREE tomato paste
1 tbsp non-iodized salt
½ tsp pepper
½ tsp dried oregano
¼ tsp dried basil
½ tsp white sugar
1 bay leaf

1. In a food processor fitted with the Steel Blade, drop garlic through feed tube while machine is running. Process until minced. Add onions and process with 3 or 4 quick on/off turns, until coarsely chopped. Do not overprocess. Brown garlic and onions slowly in hot oil in a Dutch oven or large heavy-bottomed pot for 5 minutes.
2. Insert Slicer: Slice green pepper and mushrooms, using light pressure. Add to pot and cook 2 minutes longer. Remove vegetables from pot.
3. Add ground beef to pot and brown slowly for 10 minutes, until beef loses its red color. Stir often. Add remaining ingredients to pot, stirring well to break up tomatoes. (These can also be processed for a few seconds before adding to pot.) Cover and simmer gently for about 1 ½ to 2 hours, stirring occasionally. Taste to adjust seasonings. Discard bay leaf.

Yield: 6 to 8 generous servings. Freezes well.

PEELING AND SEEDING FRESH TOMATOES FOR SAUCES:

Cut out the stem end using the point of a sharp knife. Plunge tomatoes into a pot of boiling water. Cook for 20 seconds. Pour out boiling water; immediately add cold water to cover tomatoes completely. Skins will slip off easily. Cut in half and squeeze gently to remove seeds. Coarsely chop tomatoes on the Steel Blade of the food processor using several quick on/off turns.

■ PIZZA

Homemade Pizza Sauce

3 large cloves garlic
2 large onions, cut in 2-inch chunks
28 oz can SALT-FREE tomatoes
2 – 5 ½ oz cans SALT-FREE tomato paste
1 tsp white sugar
1 tsp non-iodized salt (or to taste)
freshly ground pepper
½ tsp each dried basil and oregano
¼ tsp dried thyme
¼ tsp cayenne or red pepper flakes
1 tbsp olive oil

1. Steel Blade: Drop garlic through feed tube while machine is running.
    Process until minced. Add onions and process with 3 to 4 quick on/off
    turns, until coarsely chopped.
2. Combine all ingredients except oil in a large saucepan. Simmer uncov-
    ered for 45 minutes to 1 hour, stirring occasionally. Adjust seasonings to
    taste. Cool and transfer to a large glass jar. Add oil on top but do not stir.
    Will keep for 2 weeks in the refrigerator, or may be frozen.

Yield: About 4 cups pizza sauce, or the equivalent of four 8 oz cans.

Pizza Potato Skins
(See recipe, page 99.)

Quick Matzo Pizza
Quantities are for one pizza. Just multiply the ingredients by the number of
pizzas you need. Instead of matzo, you can substitute sliced LID-safe bread
that has been lightly toasted.

1 matzo (salt-free)
2 to 3 tbsp SALT-FREE tomato sauce or Super Salsa (see recipe, page 257)
2 tbsp chopped red and/or green pepper
2 mushrooms, sliced
4 tomato slices
non-iodized salt and pepper to taste
dried basil and/or oregano, to taste
1 tsp olive oil

1. Preheat oven to 375ºF. Line a baking sheet with foil; spray with non-stick spray. Spread matzo with sauce. Sprinkle with peppers and mushrooms. Top with tomato slices; sprinkle with seasonings. Drizzle lightly with olive oil.
2. Bake uncovered for 8 to 10 minutes (or microwave on HIGH for 1 minute), until piping hot.

Yield: 1 serving.

■ HEARTY MAIN DISHES

Basic Savory Egg White Omelet
(See recipe, page 59.)

Basic Sweet Egg White Omelet
(See recipe, page 60.)

Black Bean and Corn Casserole
Elegant enough for guests. Full of fiber, full of beans!

4 cups cooked or SALT-FREE canned black beans, well-drained
2 cups SALT-FREE canned stewed tomatoes or 2 cups Quick and Easy Tomato Sauce (see recipe, page 192)

3 tbsp honey
2 medium onions, chopped
1 green pepper, chopped
1 red pepper, chopped
¾ cup SALT-FREE canned or frozen corn niblets
½ tsp dry mustard
½ tsp each cayenne and chili powder
freshly ground pepper, to taste

1. Spray a 2 quart ovenproof casserole with non-stick spray. Combine all ingredients and mix well. Bake covered at 350°F for 45 minutes, until bubbling hot and flavors are blended. (Or microwave in a covered microsafe casserole on HIGH for 15 to 18 minutes. Stir once or twice during cooking.)

Yield: 6 servings, about 1 cup each. Freezes and/or reheats well. Delicious cold.

Cabbage Rolls

For tips on other ways to prepare cabbage leaves and make them flexible for stuffing, see Cabbage Magic (opposite).

1 head cabbage (about 3 lb)
1 lb lean ground beef or veal
2 egg whites
¾ tsp non-iodized salt
dash of pepper
1 clove garlic, minced
¼ cup raw rice
3 tbsp quick-cooking oats
19 oz can SALT-FREE tomatoes, or 6 fresh tomatoes
5 ½ oz can SALT-FREE tomato paste
⅓ cup white sugar

2 tbsp lemon juice
non-iodized salt and pepper, to taste

1. Remove 12 of the large outer leaves from cabbage, trimming away tough ribs. Place leaves in a large pot of boiling water. Remove pot from heat, cover and let stand for 10 minutes. Drain thoroughly and set aside.
2. Combine meat, egg whites, seasonings, rice, oats, and ⅓ cup juice from SALT-FREE canned tomatoes in a large bowl; mix well. Place a large spoonful of meat mixture on each cabbage leaf. Roll up, folding in ends.
3. Combine canned tomatoes, tomato paste, sugar, lemon juice, and salt and pepper to taste in a large pot; mix well. (Use the same pot to save on cleanup!) Bring to a boil over medium-high heat.
4. Carefully place cabbage rolls seam-side down in simmering sauce. Reduce heat and simmer partially covered for 1 ½ hours, until sauce has thickened slightly. Adjust seasonings to taste.

Yield: 12 cabbage rolls. Freezes and reheats well.

Cabbage Magic:

- *Large leaves are best for stuffing. Remove the core of cabbage with a sharp knife.*
- *Freezer Method: Freeze whole cabbage in a plastic bag a day or two before you need it. Remove cabbage from freezer the night before. Thaw overnight at room temperature. In the morning, the wilted leaves will separate easily.*
- *Microwave Method: Rinse cabbage but do not dry. Microwave covered on HIGH for 8 to 10 minutes, until outer leaves are pliable. Let stand covered for 3 to 4 minutes. Separate leaves. If cabbage is not flexible when you remove the last few leaves, microwave it a minute or two longer.*
- *To roll cabbage leaves more easily, pare the thick rib portion with a sharp paring knife.*
- *Leftover cabbage can be used to make Best Coleslaw (see page 135) or Cabbage Soup with Meatballs (see page 79).*

Easy BBQ Chickpea Casserole

> 4 cups cooked or canned SALT-FREE chickpeas (2 – 19 oz cans, drained and rinsed)
> 2 cups SALT-FREE canned, stewed tomatoes or 2 cups Quick and Easy Tomato Sauce (see recipe, page 192)
> 3 to 4 tbsp maple syrup or honey
> 1 medium onion, chopped
> 1 green pepper, chopped
> ½ tsp cayenne (or to taste)
> freshly ground pepper, to taste

1. Spray a 2-quart ovenproof casserole with non-stick spray. Combine all ingredients and mix well. Cover and bake at 350ºF for 1 hour. Delicious over rice.

Yield: 6 servings. Freezes and/or reheats well. Also excellent served cold.

Variations: *Add 1 cup sliced mushrooms. Season with ½ tsp each of dried basil and thyme.*

Easy Ratatouille
(See recipe, page 194.)

Easy Vegetarian Chili
You won't believe that this delicious, high-fiber chili contains no meat! Don't be deceived by the long list of ingredients. They're mostly herbs and spices. This chili is quick to prepare and tastes better the next day. Cocoa is the secret ingredient. It deepens the color and rounds out the flavor.

> 1 tbsp olive or canola oil
> 2 onions, chopped

2 green and/or red peppers, chopped

3 cloves garlic, crushed

2 cups mushrooms, sliced

2 cups cooked or canned SALT-FREE kidney beans, well-drained

2 cups cooked or canned SALT-FREE chickpeas, well-drained

½ cup bulgur or couscous, rinsed and drained

28 oz can SALT-FREE tomatoes or 6 fresh tomatoes, chopped

1 cup SALT-FREE bottled salsa (mild or medium) or Super Salsa
(see recipe, page 257)

½ cup water

1 tsp non-iodized salt (or to taste)

1 tbsp chili powder

1 tsp dried basil

½ tsp each ground pepper, dried oregano and cumin

¼ tsp cayenne (or to taste)

1 tbsp unsweetened pure cocoa powder (LID-safe)

1 tsp white sugar

1 cup SALT-FREE corn niblets (optional)

1. Conventional Method: Heat oil in a large pot. Sauté onions, peppers, and garlic for 5 minutes on medium heat. Add mushrooms and sauté 4 or 5 minutes longer. Add remaining ingredients except corn. Bring to a boil and simmer, covered, for 25 minutes, stirring occasionally. Stir in corn.

2. Microwave Method: Combine oil, onions, peppers and garlic in a 3 quart microsafe pot. Microwave covered on HIGH for 5 minutes. Add mushrooms and microwave 2 minutes longer. Add remaining ingredients except corn. Cover and microwave on HIGH for 18 to 20 minutes, stirring once or twice. Add corn. Let stand covered for 10 minutes.

Yield: 10 servings of approximately 1 cup each. Freezes and/or reheats well.

- **Gluten-Free Chili:** *If you're allergic to wheat, do not use bulgur or couscous. Instead, substitute 1 cup quinoa or millet. Rinse thoroughly and drain well. (Millet requires pre-toasting. Cook it on medium heat in a heavy-bottomed skillet for about 5 minutes, stirring constantly to prevent burning. It's ready when it gives off a toasty aroma similar to popcorn.) Add to remaining ingredients and cook as directed.*
- **Serving Suggestions:** *Serve over LID-safe noodles, rice or Basic Polenta (see recipe, page 46).*

Freeze with Ease Turkey Chili

This recipe makes a big batch, so it's perfect for freezing.

> 2 tbsp olive oil, divided
> 3 onions, chopped
> 2 cups peppers, chopped (use a mixture of red, green and yellow peppers)
> 2 cups sliced mushrooms
> 3 or 4 cloves garlic, crushed
> 3 lb ground turkey
> 19 oz can SALT-FREE red kidney beans (or 2 cups cooked beans)
> 19 oz can SALT-FREE white beans (or 2 cups cooked beans)
> 28 oz can SALT-FREE tomatoes (or 6 fresh tomatoes, finely chopped)
> 3 cups SALT-FREE tomato sauce or homemade tomato sauce
> (see recipes, pages 189 and 192)
> 2 – 5 ½ oz cans SALT-FREE tomato paste
> 19 oz can SALT-FREE tomato juice
> non-iodized salt and ground pepper, to taste
> 2 tbsp chili powder (or to taste)
> 1 tsp each dried basil and oregano (or to taste)

1. Spray a large pot with non-stick spray. Heat 1 tbsp oil on medium heat. Add onions and sauté for 5 to 7 minutes. Add peppers and mushrooms; sauté 5 minutes longer, until tender. Add a little water if veggies begin to

stick or burn. Remove veggies from pot and set aside.

2. Heat remaining oil. Add turkey and brown on medium-high heat, stirring often.

3. Rinse and drain beans. Add with remaining ingredients to pot. Simmer uncovered for 1 hour, stirring occasionally. Adjust seasonings to taste.

Yield: 15 servings. Reheats well. Freeze in meal-sized batches. Serve over LID-safe pasta or rice.

Hearty Vegetable Stew
(See recipe, page 195.)

Mini Grilled Chicken Kabobs
(See recipe, page 160.)

Old-Fashioned Hamburgers
My mother used to make these for me when I was a little girl and I loved them. The hamburgers took at least an hour to steam after they were browned, but using the microwave cuts down dramatically on time.

> 1 lb lean ground beef or veal
> 4 egg whites
> 1 tbsp water
> ¾ tsp non-iodized salt
> ¼ tsp pepper
> 1 clove garlic, minced
> ¼ cup matzo meal or quick-cooking oats
> 2 tbsp canola oil
> 1 or 2 onions, sliced

1. Combine ground beef with egg whites, water, seasonings and matzo meal or oats. Mix lightly or meat will become tough. Moisten your hands with

cold water to facilitate shaping; the mixture will be quite soft. Form meat into 5 or 6 patties.

2. Heat oil in a skillet on top of the stove. Brown patties in oil on medium-high heat, about 3 to 4 minutes per side. Transfer to a microsafe covered casserole. Brown onions quickly in pan drippings. Add to casserole.

3. Microwave covered on HIGH for 5 minutes, until juices run clear. Serve with mashed potatoes and unsalted corn niblets or peas.

Yield: 3 to 4 servings. Recipe can be doubled easily, but increase microwave cooking time to 8 to 10 minutes.

Variation: *Sauté 2 cups sliced mushrooms along with the onions.*

Oriental Vegetable Stir-Fry

2 tbsp canola oil or peanut oil
2 cloves minced garlic
1 tbsp minced fresh ginger
1 large or 2 medium onions, sliced
1 red and/or green pepper, halved, seeded and sliced
2 cups sliced mushrooms
1 cup snow peas, trimmed
2 cups bean sprouts
1 tbsp cornstarch dissolved in ¼ cup cold water
non-iodized salt and pepper, to taste
1 tsp toasted sesame oil

1. Heat oil in a wok or large skillet over medium-high heat. Add garlic and ginger and sauté for 30 seconds. Add onions, peppers and mushrooms. Stir-fry for 2 to 3 minutes, until tender-crisp. Add snow peas and bean sprouts. Stir-fry 1 minute longer.

2.	Make a well in the center of the wok or skillet. Add cornstarch/water mixture and cook until thickened, about 1 minute, stirring constantly. Season with salt, pepper and sesame oil; mix well.

Yield: 4 servings. Do not freeze.

Variations: *Add your favorite fresh or frozen veggies (e.g., broccoli florets, cauliflower florets, bok choy, cabbage, baby carrots). Use different colored peppers for added visual appeal. Leftover chicken, cut into strips or chunks, is also a nice addition.*

Quick and Spicy Turkey Meat Loaf
(See recipe, page 163.)

Red Hot Chili
(See recipe, page 174.)

Savory Shepherd's Pie

Potato Mixture:
4 potatoes, peeled and cut in chunks
boiling water to cover
non-iodized salt, to taste
2 medium onions, chopped
2 tbsp canola or olive oil
½ tsp baking powder
⅛ tsp pepper

Meat Mixture:
1 tbsp olive or canola oil
1 ½ lb lean ground beef or veal
1 tsp non-iodized salt, to taste

¼ tsp pepper
½ tsp garlic powder
2 egg whites
3 tbsp Low Iodine Homemade Ketchup (see page 183) or water
optional: paprika to garnish

Potato Mixture:

1. Cook potatoes in boiling salted water until tender. Drain well, reserving about ½ cup of the cooking water. Return pan to heat, about a minute or so, to remove excess moisture from potatoes. Mash potatoes until smooth and lump-free, adding some of the reserved cooking water.

2. While potatoes are cooking, sauté onions in 2 tbsp hot oil in a large skillet until golden, about 5 minutes. Add onions to mashed potatoes along with baking powder. (Don't bother washing the skillet.) Season with salt and pepper to taste; mix well. Set aside.

Meat Mixture and Assembly:

3. Heat 1 tbsp oil in the same skillet in which you sautéed the onions. Add meat and cook over medium heat about 4 to 5 minutes, mashing it to keep it crumbly. When meat has lost its red color, add seasonings, egg whites and ketchup or water. Mix well.

4. Spread meat mixture in a greased 1 ½ quart casserole. Top with potato mixture. (If desired, make an attractive design with a fork and sprinkle with a little paprika.) Bake in a preheated 375ºF oven for 45 minutes, until golden.

Yield: 4 to 6 servings. Reheats and/or freezes well.

Variation: *Top meat mixture with 1 cup drained SALT-FREE corn niblets (or peas and carrots) before topping it with the potato mixture.*

Stuffed Peppers

The meat and rice are cooked separately, then combined and stuffed into the partially cooked peppers for a brief cooking and blending of flavors.

Ground Meat and Peppers:

1 lb lean ground beef or veal
1 small onion, chopped
⅓ cup SALT-FREE canned tomato sauce or Fresh Tomato Sauce
(see recipe, page 189)
3 tbsp quick-cooking oats
1 cup cooked white rice
¾ tsp non-iodized salt
dash of pepper
1 clove garlic, crushed
¼ tsp dried oregano
4 medium green or red peppers

Sauce Mixture:

1 cup additional SALT-FREE tomato sauce
1 tbsp honey
non-iodized salt, to taste
dash of pepper and oregano

Ground Meat and Peppers:

1. Combine ground beef or veal and onion in a 1-quart microsafe casserole. Microwave uncovered on HIGH for 5 minutes, until no pink remains, stirring once or twice during cooking. Add ⅓ cup SALT-FREE tomato sauce, oats, rice, salt, pepper, garlic, and oregano. Mix well.
2. Cut peppers in half. Remove membranes and seeds. Arrange cut-side up in an oblong Pyrex casserole. Cover with parchment paper. Microwave on high for 4 to 5 minutes, until tender-crisp. Drain. Spoon in filling.

Sauce Mixture and Assembly:

3.   Combine remaining 1 cup of tomato sauce with honey, salt, pepper, and oregano. Spoon into peppers. Cover with parchment paper. (Can be prepared in advance up to this point and refrigerated.)

4.   Microwave on HIGH for 10 to 12 minutes, until peppers are tender, rotating the casserole halfway through cooking. (Or bake covered in a preheated 375ºF oven for 30 minutes.) Let stand covered for 5 minutes. Serve with a green salad, unsalted corn niblets, and crusty rolls.

Yield: 4 servings. Can be frozen.

CHAPTER SIX

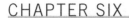

DINNERS
THE MOST INTERESTING MEALS

WHAT'S INSIDE

121

■ SOUPS

Avocado Cucumber Soup
(See recipe, page 78.)

Beef Barley Soup
(See recipe, page 79.)

Black Bean Soup
Excellent, easy, and full of fiber! Impress your guests with its wonderful South American flavor.

> 2 cups dried black beans, rinsed and drained
> 6 cups cold water (for soaking the beans)
> 2 onions, coarsely chopped
> 4 cloves garlic, minced
> 4 stalks celery, coarsely chopped
> 1 tbsp olive oil
> 4 large carrots, coarsely chopped
> 1 tsp dried basil
> ½ tsp dried red pepper flakes
> 1 tsp cumin (to taste)
> 8 cups SALT-FREE chicken broth or broth from Free Chicken Soup or Vegetable Broth (see recipes, pages 83 and 134)
> non-iodized salt and ground pepper, to taste

1. Soak beans overnight in cold water. Drain and rinse well. Discard soaking water.
2. Prepare vegetables (this can be done in the processor). Heat oil in a large soup pot. Add onions, garlic, and celery. Sauté for 5 or 6 minutes on medium heat, until golden. If necessary, add a little water or broth to prevent sticking.

3. Add drained beans, carrots, basil, red pepper flakes, cumin and broth. Do not add salt and pepper until beans are cooked. Cover partially and simmer until beans are tender, about 2 hours, stirring occasionally. Purée part or all of the soup, if desired. If too thick, thin with water or broth. Add non-iodized salt and ground pepper to taste.

Yield: 10 servings. Freezes well.

Chef's Secrets:

- *Soak and drain beans as directed in Step 1. Place soaked beans in a storage container and pop them in the freezer for up to 2 months. When you want to make soup, just add the frozen beans to the pot. No need to defrost them first. (You can use this trick with any kind of beans!)*
- *If you have time, presoak a batch of black beans, then cook them for 1 ½ to 2 hours, until tender. Drain, cool and freeze. When you want soup, add 3 to 4 cups of frozen cooked beans to the soup pot without thawing. Your soup will be ready in just half an hour!*
- *Are you afraid to eat beans because you're worried about possible embarrassing moments? If you presoak beans, and then discard the soaking water, you'll eliminate the problem of gas! As an extra precaution, rinse the beans again thoroughly after presoaking them.*
- *Serving Tip: For an elegant touch, garnish each serving with a spoonful of homemade Super Salsa or chopped Roasted Red Peppers (for recipes, see pages 257 and 259).*

Cabbage Soup with Meatballs
(See recipe, page 79.)

Chicken, Lima Bean, and Barley Soup

Roz Brown and I have been best friends for more years than we both care to count. This is one of her recipe treasures. Her daughter, Stephanie, asks for this soup whenever she visits from England. She calls this fiber-full soup "a meal in a bowl."

2 cups dried lima beans

6 cups cold water (for soaking the beans)

1 chicken, cut up (about 3 lb)

12 cups water (approximately)

2 onions

4 stalks celery

4 or 5 large carrots

3 parsnips

½ turnip, if desired

2 tsp non-iodized salt

½ tsp ground pepper

¾ cup pearl barley, rinsed and drained

3 or 4 potatoes, peeled and cut in small chunks

¼ cup fresh dill, chopped

1. Rinse beans and place them in a bowl. Cover with cold water and let them soak.

2. Remove skin and excess fat from chicken. Place chicken in a large soup pot. Add 12 cups water and bring to a boil. Remove scum. Add onions, celery, carrots, parsnips and turnip (no need to chop them). Season with non-iodized salt and pepper.

3. Simmer partly covered for 1 ½ hours, until chicken is tender. Remove chicken and vegetables from pot and let them cool.

4. Rinse and drain the soaked beans. Add beans and barley to broth. Bring to a boil, reduce heat, and simmer covered for about 1 hour. Add potatoes and cook 10 to 15 minutes longer, until tender.

5.   Meanwhile, remove chicken from bones. Cut into bite-sized pieces. Slice the cooked carrots. (Roz discards the celery, turnips, and parsnips, but they can be added to the soup.) Add chicken and carrots (and remaining cooked veggies, if desired) to the pot. Add dill and simmer 10 to 15 minutes longer. Adjust seasonings to taste.

Yield: 12 generous servings. Freezes and/or reheats well. Leftover soup will get very thick and will need to be thinned with a little chicken broth or water when reheated.

Chicken Spaghetti Soup
(See recipe, page 80.)

Chilled Beet Soup
(See recipe, page 82.)

Country Vegetable Soup
The microwaved version of this low-calorie soup is made without fat.

    1 large onion, chopped
    1 stalk celery, chopped
    1 large leek, thinly sliced
    1 tbsp oil, optional
    1 tbsp water
    2 medium potatoes, peeled and chopped
    2 large carrots, peeled and chopped
    1 medium zucchini, chopped
    1 cup broccoli or cauliflower, cut up
    28 oz can SALT-FREE tomatoes
    4 cups hot water
    2 tsp non-iodized salt
    freshly ground pepper, to taste

½ tsp dried thyme
½ tsp dried basil
2 tbsp fresh parsley, minced

1. Microwave Method: Place onion, celery, leeks and water in a 3-quart microsafe casserole. Microwave covered on HIGH until tender, about 6 to 7 minutes, stirring once. Add remaining ingredients except parsley. Microwave covered on HIGH for 20 to 25 minutes, until veggies are tender. Adjust seasonings to taste. Garnish with parsley.
2. Stovetop Method: Heat 1 tbsp oil in a large soup pot. Add onion, celery and leeks. Sauté for 7 to 8 minutes, until golden. Add water as needed to prevent sticking. Add remaining ingredients except parsley. Bring to a boil and simmer covered until veggies are tender, about 35 to 40 minutes. Adjust seasonings to taste. Garnish with parsley.

Yield: 7 to 8 servings. Freezes and/or reheats well.

Free Chicken Soup
(See recipe, page 83.)

CHEF'S STOCK SECRETS:
- All or part of the vegetables can be processed in the processor or a blender, and then stirred back into the broth for a puréed vegetable soup.
- Never store hot soups (or any hot foods) in plastic containers! (The plasticizers can melt into the food.) Instead, store foods in heat-resistant glass or ceramic containers.
- Pretend Vegetable Broth: Save the cooking water from vegetables and refrigerate or freeze it until needed. I use the cooking water from veggies like carrots, peas, frozen mixed vegetables, spinach, or Swiss chard. (Don't use the water from starchy vegetables or potatoes.) I also like to save the soaking water from dried mushrooms. Any or all of these can be used

when vegetable broth is called for in a recipe. They'll add flavor without adding fat!

- A handful or two of any of the following can be added to the broth: eggplant, tomatoes, Swiss chard, spinach leaves, or any other odds and ends of veggies.
- Dried mushrooms, such as shiitake, morels, or Chinese mushrooms, add flavor to any broth. Soak them first in hot water for 20 to 30 minutes to rehydrate, then add both mushrooms and soaking liquid to broth and cook as desired.
- Many chefs freeze the trimmings from vegetables to make broth (e.g., onions, leeks, carrots, celery, mushrooms). When they have enough, they place them in a pot (no need to defrost them), cover with water, add a couple of cloves of garlic, some herbs, and a bay leaf. Simmer everything for 45 minutes and voila, almost instant broth!

Garden Vegetable Soup

3 onions, quartered
1 green pepper, cut in 1 inch chunks
½ small cabbage (about 3 cups grated)
3 stalks celery
3 carrots, scraped and trimmed
2 potatoes, peeled
3 tbsp olive oil
2 tbsp flour
2 quarts boiling water or broth from Free Chicken Soup
(see recipe, page 83)
non-iodized salt and ground pepper, to taste

1. Steel Blade (see "Variation" on next page): Add half of onions and process with 3 or 4 quick on/off turns. Empty bowl and repeat with remaining onions. Empty bowl and repeat with green pepper.

2.   Slicer: Cut cabbage, celery, carrots, and potatoes to fit feed tube. Slice, emptying bowl as necessary.
3.   Heat oil on medium heat in a large soup pot or Dutch oven. Add vegetables and cook on medium heat for 6 to 8 minutes, stirring occasionally. Sprinkle flour over and cook 1 minute longer, stirring constantly. Add boiling water (or broth) and seasonings. Cover and bring to a boil. Reduce heat and simmer covered for about 1 hour, stirring occasionally.

Yield: 8 servings. May be frozen.

Variation: *Using the Steel Blade, process separately with on/off turns to chop coarsely: 1 cup green beans, 1 cup wax beans, 2 stalks broccoli. Add to soup along with ½ small head cauliflower (broken into small florets) plus a 28 oz can of SALT-FREE tomatoes.*

Homemade Beef or Veal Broth

This easy, tasty broth can be used in the same way as chicken broth. Roasting the bones gives the broth a richer taste.

   4 to 5 lb beef or veal bones
   2 large onions (rinsed; peeling is not necessary)
   3 or 4 stalks celery
   4 to 6 large carrots
   1 bay leaf
   12 cups water (approximately)
   2 or 3 whole cloves garlic
   ½ cup fresh dill sprigs (do not chop)
   non-iodized salt and ground pepper, to taste

1.   Place bones in a roasting pan and roast uncovered at 400ºF for about an hour, until nicely browned.

2. Transfer bones to a large pot. Add onions, celery, carrots, and bay leaf. Add enough water to completely cover the bones and vegetables. Bring to a boil and skim well. Reduce heat and simmer partially covered, adding hot water as needed to keep ingredients covered. Simmer broth for 2 to 3 hours.

3. Add garlic and dill; simmer 10 to 15 minutes longer. If desired, season with non-iodized salt and pepper.

4. Cool broth slightly. Strain, discarding bones and vegetables. Refrigerate broth overnight. Lift off and discard any hardened fat. Ladle the broth into 1 or 2 cup freezer containers, discarding the layer of cloudy broth at the bottom of the soup.

Yield: About 9 cups. Broth can be frozen for 3 or 4 months.

MORE SOUPER SECRETS!

- When cooking soup, should you keep a lid on it? If the soup is completely covered, it may boil over and make a mess. If you cook it completely uncovered, too much evaporation may take place. Hearty soups, such as bean and barley or minestrone, can become thick and stick to the bottom of the pot. My solution is to cover the pot partially. This makes it easier to control the amount of evaporation that takes place, and still produce a flavorful soup.
- Meat-based broths can be used to make a variety of quick and easy soups. Add whatever fresh or frozen veggies you may have on hand, so long as they're salt-free (e.g., chopped celery, carrots, potatoes, parsnips, corn niblets, cabbage, zucchini, salt-free canned tomatoes). Salt-free beans or legumes can also be added. Cook until tender. Season to taste.
- Choose your favorite herbs (e.g., thyme, basil, dill). If using dried herbs, add them at the beginning of cooking. If using fresh herbs, add near the end of cooking and let soup simmer a few minutes to release the flavor. Enjoy!

> • For convenience, freeze homemade broth in small quantities in ice cube trays. Once frozen, transfer to an airtight storage container or a heavy-duty freezer bag. Use to flavor sauces, vegetables, and casseroles. Each cube contains about 2 tbsp broth.

Jewish Soup Dumplings

These light, fluffy dumplings are also called "matzo balls." If making a double recipe, you can use an 8-ounce carton of egg whites, which is the equivalent of 4 whole eggs.

½ cup matzo meal
½ tsp non-iodized salt
⅛ tsp white pepper
¼ tsp parsley flakes
pinch of powdered ginger, if desired
4 egg whites
2 tbsp oil
2 tbsp cold water
about 2 quarts water, with 1 tsp non-iodized salt added

1. In a mixing bowl or food processor, combine matzo meal, salt, pepper, parsley flakes, and ginger, if using. Add egg whites and oil; mix well. Blend in water. Cover and refrigerate for at least 30 minutes. (Can be prepared up to a day in advance.)
2. In a large pot, heat salted water until boiling. Wet your hands before shaping each matzo ball; form into 1-inch balls. Drop gently into boiling water. Cover, simmer over very low heat for 30 to 40 minutes.
3. To serve, remove matzo balls carefully from hot liquid with a slotted spoon and add them to soup bowls. Ladle hot soup over matzo balls.

Yield: About 10 soup dumplings/matzo balls. May be frozen in soup. You can also place them on a tray, freeze them, then transfer to freezer storage bags.

Delicious in Free Chicken Soup or Garden Vegetable Soup (see recipes, page 83 and 127).

LID Soup Dumplings

2 egg whites
½ cup water
1 cup all-purpose flour
½ tsp non-iodized salt
½ tsp baking powder

1.   Blend egg whites, water, flour, salt, and baking powder until smooth. Drop from a spoon into simmering soup. Cover and simmer 5 minutes.

Luscious Lentil Soup

Easy and healthy! Although it takes about the same amount of time to microwave this soup as to cook it on top of the stove, it never sticks to the bottom of the pot when you microwave it. Your food processor will chop the vegetables 1-2-3.

1 large onion, chopped
4 cloves garlic, minced
1 tbsp olive or canola oil
1 cup brown or red lentils, rinsed and drained
1 stalk celery, chopped
28 oz can SALT-FREE tomatoes (or 5 to 6 fresh ripe tomatoes, chopped)
5 cups water (approximately)
1 bay leaf
1 ½ tsp non-iodized salt (to taste)
½ tsp pepper
1 tsp dried basil or dill (or 1 tbsp fresh)
juice of ½ lemon (about 1 ½ tbsp)
¼ cup fresh parsley, minced

1. Microwave Method: In a 3-quart microsafe pot, combine onion, garlic and oil. Microwave uncovered on HIGH for 4 minutes. Add remaining ingredients except lemon juice and parsley; mix well. Microwave covered on HIGH for 1 hour, until lentils are tender. Stir once or twice during cooking. If boiling too much, reduce power to MEDIUM (50%). If too thick, add some boiling water. Add lemon juice. Adjust seasonings to taste. Let stand at least 10 minutes to allow flavors to blend. Discard bay leaf. Garnish with parsley.

2. Conventional Method: Heat oil in a large soup pot. Add onions; sauté on medium heat until golden, about 4 or 5 minutes. Add garlic and sauté 2 or 3 minutes longer. Add 2 or 3 tbsp water if vegetables begin to stick. Add remaining ingredients except lemon juice and parsley. Bring to a boil, reduce heat and simmer partially covered for 1 hour, until lentils are tender, stirring occasionally. Thin with a little hot water if too thick. Add lemon juice. Adjust seasonings to taste. Discard bay leaf. Garnish with parsley.

Yield: 8 to 10 servings. Tastes even better the next day! Freezes well.

Variations: *For more fiber, add 2 or 3 carrots, coarsely chopped, to the sautéed onions. Proceed as directed. Add 1 cup cooked pasta or rice to the cooked soup. For a Middle Eastern flavor, substitute coriander (cilantro) for basil or dill.*

Mushroom Barley Soup
(See recipe, page 84.)

Potato Mushroom Soup
(See recipe, page 84.)

Purée of Red Pepper Soup
(See recipe, page 85.)

Quick Gazpacho

(See recipe, page 86.)

The Best Chicken Soup

I make my chicken soup with lots of carrots because they add wonderful flavor. Also, I love carrots! When I had pneumonia, my friend Doris Fink nursed me back to health by adding a red pepper to the soup. Since I did recover, I now use her trick when making chicken soup. I also add garlic and lots of dill. Chicken soup is really marvelous for colds and flu. Also, it tastes terrific!

3 lb chicken, cut up
8 cups water (approximately)
non-iodized salt, to taste
½ tsp pepper
7 or 8 carrots
4 stalks celery
2 onions (or 1 onion and 1 leek)
1 red pepper, cored, seeded, and cut up
2 cloves garlic
½ cup fresh dill sprigs (do not chop)

1. Trim excess fat from chicken. To remove excess salt from Kosher chicken, soak it in cold water for ½ hour. Rinse and drain well. Place chicken in a narrow, deep soup pot. Add water. (It should cover the chicken completely.) Add non-iodized salt and ground pepper. Bring to a boil.
2. Remove scum completely. Add carrots, celery, onions, and red pepper. Cover partially and simmer gently for 1 to 1 ½ hours.
3. Add garlic and dill. Simmer soup 10 to 15 minutes longer. Adjust seasonings to taste.

4.   Cool completely. Strain soup. Discard skin and fat from chicken (see page 83). Discard all veggies except the carrots. Refrigerate soup overnight. Discard hardened fat from surface of soup.

Yield: 6 to 8 servings. Reheats and/or freezes well.

THERE'S ALWAYS ROOM FOR SOUP!
- Serve soup with LID-safe noodles, rice, orzo, kasha, matzo farfel or Homemade Matzo Balls (for recipe, see page 130). Add a piece of carrot to each bowl; garnish with fresh dill.
- Serve boiled chicken as a main dish, or add pieces of cut-up chicken to the soup. Cooked chicken can be used for chicken salad, casseroles, sandwiches, or crêpes.
- Jewish chicken soup is traditionally flavored with dill and the veggies are cooked in large chunks. French chefs add thyme and bay leaf to their soup, and they dice the vegetables neatly. Vive la différence!

Vegetable Barley Soup
(See recipe, page 87.)

Vegetable Broth ("Almost Chicken Soup")
This recipe makes an excellent substitution for commercial vegetable broth, which is loaded with salt.

2 large onions (or 1 onion and 1 leek, including about 2 inches of green top)
7 or 8 carrots
4 stalks celery
1 red pepper
1 cup mushrooms (optional)
9 cups cold water
non-iodized salt, to taste

ground pepper, to taste
3 cloves garlic, peeled
½ cup fresh dill sprigs (do not chop)

1. Clean vegetables and cut them into large chunks. Place all ingredients except garlic and dill in a large soup pot. Water should cover vegetables by no more than 1 inch. Bring to a boil. Reduce heat, cover partially, and simmer for 30 minutes.
2. Add garlic and dill and cook 10 minutes longer. Strain and serve with Homemade Matzo Balls (see recipe, page 130), LID Soup Dumplings (see page 131), matzo farfel, LID-safe noodles or rice.

Yield: About 8 cups. Can be frozen for up to 3 months.

■ SALADS

Balsamic Salad Splash
(See recipe, page 88.)

Best Coleslaw
This tried and true recipe lives up to its name, it's a winner! The food processor speeds up preparation. I prefer using young cabbage, if possible.

Coleslaw Mixture:
1 head cabbage (about 3 lb)
3 medium carrots, peeled and trimmed
2 cloves garlic, peeled
3 green onions, cut in 2-inch pieces
1 green pepper, cut in long, narrow strips

Marinade:
1 cup white vinegar
½ cup white sugar (see Note)

¾ cup canola oil
1 tsp non-iodized salt
¼ tsp pepper

1. Slicer: Cut cabbage into wedges to fit feed tube. Discard core. Slice, using very light pressure. If you prefer a finer texture, you can use the Grater (use firm pressure). If too thick, chop in batches on the Steel Blade, using quick on/off pulses.
2. Place cabbage in a large bowl.
3. Grater: Cut carrots to fit feed tube crosswise. Grate, using firm pressure. Add to cabbage.
4. Steel Blade: Drop garlic and green onions through feed tube while machine is running. Process until minced.
5. Slicer: Stack green pepper vertically in feed tube. Slice, using light pressure. Add to cabbage mixture.
6. Combine ingredients for marinade in a saucepan and bring to a boil. Pour hot marinade over coleslaw mixture and toss well. Transfer to a large jar or bowl, cover tightly and refrigerate.

Yield: 12 to 16 servings. Do not freeze.

Note: *This coleslaw will keep about 3 to 4 weeks in the refrigerator without becoming soggy. For calorie counters, eliminate all or part of the sugar.*

Israeli Salad
(See recipe, page 90.)

Italiano Dressing
(See recipe, page 91.)

Marinated Bean Salad
(See recipe, page 91.)

Orange Balsamic Vinaigrette
(See recipe, page 93.)

Red Cabbage Coleslaw
The boiled dressing transforms the cabbage into a beautiful, brilliant magenta color.

> 1 medium red cabbage, cored and thinly sliced (about 8 cups)
> 4 green onions, thinly sliced
> 1 medium carrot, grated
> 2 tbsp canola oil
> ¼ cup red or white wine vinegar (also excellent with raspberry or balsamic vinegar)
> 2 tbsp white sugar
> non-iodized salt and ground pepper, to taste

1. Combine vegetables in a large mixing bowl. (A food processor will save time when preparing the vegetables.)
2. In a medium saucepan, combine oil, vinegar and white sugar. Bring to a boil. (Or combine in a 2-cup Pyrex measure and microwave uncovered for 45 seconds.)
3. Pour hot dressing over vegetables. Mix well. Add salt and pepper to taste. Refrigerate to blend flavors.

Yield: 12 servings. Leftovers keep 3 to 4 days in the refrigerator.

Simply Basic Vinaigrette
(See recipe, page 93.)

Tomato, Onion, and Pepper Salad
(See recipe, page 94.)

■ SIDE DISHES

Apricot Candied Carrots

2 lb carrots, scraped and trimmed
½ cup boiling water
dash of non-iodized salt
½ cup apricot jam
8 marshmallows

1.   Slicer: Cut carrots to fit feed tube. Slice, using firm pressure.
2.   Combine boiling water, salt, and jam in a saucepan. Add carrots, cover and cook about 15 to 20 minutes, until tender. Remove cover and let liquid boil down to a depth of half an inch. Add marshmallows; stir until dissolved and carrots are nicely glazed.

Yield: 6 to 8 servings. May be frozen.

Note: *This dish reheats very well. You may reheat it in the oven or microwave, if desired. If you prefer a sweeter taste, add 2 to 3 tbsp honey along with the marshmallows.*

ASPARAGUS MICROWAVE TIPS
- Pencil thin asparuagus is best. Delicious hot or cold.
- Break woody portion from asparagus stems and discard. Rinse asparagus under cold running water. Do not dry. Arrange in an oblong microsafe casserole with stalks towards the outside of the casserole and tips meeting in the center. Cover casserole with parchment paper that you've placed briefly under running water to make it flexible, so that it can be molded around the dish easily.
- Microwave until tender-crisp (see next tip). Let stand covered for 2 minutes. Season as desired.

- ½ lb asparagus (1 to 2 servings) will take 3 to 4 minutes on HIGH to microwave. 1 ½ lb takes 6 to 8 minutes to cook and serves 4.
- If I want to cook just a few stalks of asparagus for myself, I rinse them with cold water, then stand them with the tips pointing upwards in a glass measuring cup. Cover the asparagus and measuring cup loosely with cooking parchment and microwave on HIGH for 1 to 2 minutes, until bright green. Let stand covered for 1 minute.

Asparagus Vinaigrette
Elegant and easy!

1 ½ lb asparagus
½ cup olive oil
3 tbsp wine vinegar
½ tsp dry mustard
1 clove crushed garlic
non-iodized salt and pepper, to taste
2 hard-cooked egg whites, chopped (discard yolks)
½ of a red pepper, chopped

1. Prepare asparagus as directed in Asparagus Mircowave Tips (preceding). Microwave covered on HIGH for 6 minutes, until tender-crisp. Arrange on a serving plate.
2. Combine olive oil, vinegar, mustard, garlic, salt, and pepper in a mixing bowl. Blend with a whisk. Drizzle over asparagus. (Any leftover dressing can be refrigerated for another time.)
3. Garnish asparagus with alternating bands of egg white and red peppers. Chill before serving.

Yield: 4 to 6 servings. Do not freeze.

Green Beans Almondine

1 lb fresh green beans
 boiling water to cover, salted with non-iodized salt
1 onion, halved
2 tbsp olive oil
¼ cup slivered almonds
non-iodized salt and pepper, to taste

1. Slicer: Wash and trim beans. Cut in half to fit feed tube crosswise. Pack beans tightly so that they're lying on their sides in the feed tube. Slice, using very firm pressure. Repeat with remaining beans in as many batches as necessary.
2. Place in a saucepan with boiling salted water. Cover and cook on medium heat for 5 to 7 minutes, until nearly tender. Drain well.
3. Steel Blade: Process onion with 2 or 3 quick on/off turns, until coarsely chopped. Pour oil into a skillet. Add onion and sauté lightly. Stir in almonds and beans. Cook for 2 to 3 minutes, stirring to mix. Season to taste.

Yield: 4 servings. May be prepared in advance and reheated in the microwave, but best served fresh.

Honey-Glazed Carrots

This is a terrific company dish. For a smaller family, make half the amount. Leftovers reheat beautifully.

4 lb carrots, peeled and sliced
2 tbsp cornstarch
1 cup orange juice
½ to ¾ cup liquid honey (to taste)
¼ cup orange marmalade or apricot preserves

3 tbsp lemon juice
non-iodized salt and ground pepper, to taste

1. Cook carrots in boiling salted water to cover until tender, about 15 minutes. Drain off most of the water, leaving about 1 inch in the bottom of the pot. Dissolve cornstarch in orange juice. Add to carrots. Stir in honey, marmalade, and lemon juice. Season to taste with non-iodized salt and ground pepper.
2. Bring mixture to a boil, stirring gently. Transfer to a sprayed ovenproof or microsafe casserole. (Can be prepared up to this point, covered and refrigerated.)
3. Bake uncovered in a preheated 350°F oven for 25 minutes (or microwave covered on HIGH for 10 minutes), stirring once or twice.

Yield: 12 servings. Freezes and/or reheats well.

Microwave Corn on the Cob

There are several methods of cooking corn in the microwave. All methods work well. Use a microsafe dinner plate or oblong microsafe casserole. Cooking time can vary depending on size of corn and freshness.

Method 1: Peel the husks back but don't detatch them. They'll act as a natural covering for the corn. Remove the silk. Rinse corn under cold water and shake off excess moisture. Recover with husks. Arrange on a plate or in a casserole. (Cooking time is a few seconds longer because the husks absorb some of the microwave energy.)

Method 2: Remove husks and silk. Rinse corn under cold water and shake off excess moisture. Use waxed paper or cooking parchment to wrap each individual cob. Twist ends like a firecracker to seal. Arrange corn on plate or in casserole. (Or, instead of wrapping each ear of corn individually, just cover the dish with parchment or waxed paper.)

To Cook: Microwave on HIGH, allowing 2 to 3 minutes per ear of corn. Re-arrange corn at half time if your microwave oven cooks unevenly. (I allow 2 to 2 ½ minutes per ear if cooking 4 or more.) Let stand 2 to 3 minutes to complete cooking. Unwrap, brush with olive oil and sprinkle with non-iodized salt and pepper. Cajun Seasoning or Seasoned Salt also make tasty toppings (see recipes, page 243).

BBQ Corn: Microwave corn on HIGH for 2 minutes per ear, then unwrap carefully and transfer immediately to the hot BBQ. Grill for several minutes, turning often, to acquire that just-roasted flavor.

Minted Peas with Red Peppers

Green peas are more nutritious than green beans! They contain vitamins A and C and are high in fiber. Fresh basil can be substituted for mint.

> 10 oz package frozen SALT-FREE green peas
> 2 tsp olive oil
> 4 green onions (white part only), chopped
> 1 red pepper, chopped
> 1 to 2 tbsp chopped fresh mint
> non-iodized salt and ground pepper, to taste
> 1 tbsp fresh lime or lemon juice

1. Bring a saucepan of water to a boil. Add peas and simmer 3 to 4 minutes, until tender-crisp. Drain and rinse well under cold water to stop the cooking process. Set aside.
2. Pour olive oil into a non-stick skillet. Add green onions and red pepper. Sauté for 3 or 4 minutes, until softened. Add peas and mint. Cook for 1 to 2 minutes, just until heated through. Add seasonings and lime juice. Serve immediately.

Yield: 3 to 4 servings.

Oriental Vegetable Stir Fry

(See recipe, page 116.)

Oven Roasted Garlic Potatoes

Yummy, yet so easy.

> 4 large baking potatoes, cut into eighths (peel if desired)
> non-iodized salt and ground pepper, to taste
> 1 tsp dried rosemary, crushed
> 1 tsp paprika (preferably Hungarian)
> 3 to 4 cloves garlic, crushed (to taste)
> 1 tbsp olive oil

1. Preheat oven to 400ºF. Spray a 2 quart ovenproof casserole with non-stick spray. Sprinkle potatoes with seasonings, garlic, and olive oil. Rub mixture over potatoes to coat evenly. Cover casserole with foil.
2. Bake at 400ºF for 35 to 40 minutes. Remove foil and roast uncovered 30 minutes longer, stirring occasionally. Potatoes should be fork-tender, yet golden and crispy.

Yield: 4 to 5 servings. Do not freeze.

Pizza Potato Skins

(See recipe, page 99.)

Rice Pea-laf with Peppers

Prepare Minted Peas with Red Peppers as directed (see recipe, page 142). Combine with 3 cups of cooked white or brown basmati rice. Add non-iodized salt and ground pepper to taste.

Roasted Carrots

(See recipe, page 97.)

Roasted Garlic Mashed Potatoes

Thanks to Gloria Schachter for this great recipe. Guaranteed to keep the vampires away!

> 1 head of Roasted Garlic (see recipe, page 225)
> 4 or 5 potatoes, peeled and cut into chunks
> 1 tbsp olive oil
> ¾ tsp non-iodized salt
> freshly ground pepper, to taste

1. Roast garlic as directed. Cook potatoes in lightly salted water (using non-iodized salt) until soft, about 20 minutes. Drain off most of the water, reserving ½ cup. Return pot with potatoes to the heat and let them dry for a minute or two to evaporate excess moisture. Remove from heat.
2. Mash potatoes with a potato masher or potato ricer. Squeeze the garlic cloves into potatoes and mash well. Gradually beat in the reserved cooking water a little at a time until light and creamy. Add oil, salt, and pepper.

Yield: 4 servings. Do not freeze. These can be reheated in the microwave.

Saucy Lemon Zucchini

1 lb zucchini, ends trimmed
1 onion, quartered
1 clove garlic, crushed
2 tbsp olive oil
½ tsp non-iodized salt
⅛ tsp pepper
¼ tsp dried basil
1 tbsp white sugar
1 ½ tbsp lemon juice
2 tsp cornstarch, dissolved in 2 tbsp cold water

1. Insert Slicer in processor. Slice zucchini and onions, using medium pressure. Add to casserole. Add garlic, olive oil, salt, pepper, basil, sugar, and lemon juice. Mix well.
2. Cover and microwave on HIGH for 5 to 6 minutes, stirring at half time. Zucchini should be almost translucent.
3. Stir in cornstarch mixture and microwave uncovered on HIGH 2 minutes longer, until sauce is thickened and zucchini is piping hot. Stir and serve immediately.

Yield: 3 to 4 servings.

Squished Squash

Nutrient-packed, rich in beta-carotene and folic acid, this dish is potassi-yummy!

2 acorn squash or 1 butternut squash*
1 to 2 tbsp olive oil
non-iodized salt and ground pepper, to taste
½ tsp ground cinnamon
½ tsp ground nutmeg

1. Preheat oven to 375ºF. Cut squash in half crosswise. (To cut it in half easily, microwave it first for 2 to 3 minutes on HIGH.) Place cut-side down on a sprayed non-stick baking pan. Bake uncovered until tender, about 50 to 60 minutes.
2. Cool slightly, then scoop out and discard seeds and stringy pulp from squash. Scoop out the flesh from squash into a bowl and mash together with olive oil and seasonings. Reheat before serving.

Yield: 4 servings. Do not freeze.

Winter varieties include acorn, buttercup, butternut, Hubbard, pumpkin, spaghetti, and turban squash. They don't need refrigeration, they can be stored at room temperature for about a month.

Variation: *Instead of roasting squash, here's how to microwave it: Pierce squash in several places with a sharp knife. Place on a microsafe rack and microwave on HIGH, allowing 5 to 7 minutes per lb. Turn squash over halfway through cooking. Total cooking time will be 12 to 14 minutes. Then continue as directed in Step 2.*

Tasty Green Beans

The food processor makes French-style green beans in a flash. If you don't have a processor, slice green beans diagonally into thin slices.

1 lb fresh green beans
boiling water to cover, salted with non-iodized salt
2 tbsp olive oil
non-iodized salt and pepper, to taste
1 tsp fresh lemon juice

1. Insert Slicer in processor. Wash and trim beans. Cut in half to fit feed tube crosswise. Pack beans tightly so that they're lying on their sides in the feed tube. Slice, using very firm pressure. Repeat with remaining beans in as many batches as necessary.
2. Place in saucepan with boiling salted water. Cover and cook on medium heat for 5 to 7 minutes, until tender but still slightly crunchy. Drain well. Combine with remaining ingredients.

Yield: 4 servings. Best served fresh, but may be prepared in advance.

Vegetable Stuffing
Kind to the calorie conscious!

2 onions
1 zucchini, unpeeled
2 large carrots, peeled
4 egg whites
1 cup matzo meal
¾ tsp non-iodized salt
freshly ground pepper
⅛ tsp dried oregano
⅛ tsp dried basil
½ tsp paprika

1. Insert grater in food processor. Cut vegetables to fit feed tube. Grate onions and zucchini, using medium pressure. Grate carrots, using firm pressure.

2. Push vegetables to one side and insert Steel Blade in processor bowl. Add remaining ingredients and process with several quick on/off turns until mixed, about 8 to 10 seconds. Do not overprocess.

Yield: Enough for a 10 or 12 pound turkey, or a large veal brisket, or 2 small chickens. Remove stuffing from poultry or meat if you plan to freeze it, and wrap separately for freezing.

Variation: *For stuffing casserole, bake stuffing mixture separately in a covered greased casserole at 325ºF for 40 to 45 minutes.*

Yum-Yum Potato Wedgies
(See recipe, page 101.)

■ POULTRY

Breaded Chicken Fillets

6 single chicken breasts, skinned and boned
1 cup matzo meal
1 tsp non-iodized salt
¼ tsp pepper
¼ tsp garlic powder
½ tsp Italian seasoning (or a mixture of dried basil and oregano)
½ tsp paprika
2 egg whites
1 tbsp water
oil for frying

1. Wash and dry chicken breasts well.
2. Combine matzo meal with seasonings in a pie plate or large heavy-duty plastic bag; mix well.
3. Blend egg whites with water in a pie plate. Dip chicken pieces first into

egg mixture, then into crumbs.

4. Brown in hot oil over medium heat on both sides until golden brown. Total cooking time is about 6 to 8 minutes. Do not crowd frying pan. Drain well on paper towels.

Yield: 4 to 6 servings. May be frozen. Allow for seconds! Delicious with mashed potatoes and a big garden salad or steamed broccoli.

Note: *May be browned in advance and reheated uncovered at 400ºF for about 10 minutes.*

Cantonese-Style Almond Chicken

4 boneless, skinless single chicken breasts
2 cups mushrooms
1 medium onion, halved
2 tbsp peanut or canola oil
1 tsp minced garlic
1 tbsp minced fresh ginger
1 cup frozen peas
¼ cup SALT-FREE chicken broth or broth from Free Chicken Soup (see recipe, page 83)
1 tsp toasted sesame oil
1 tbsp cornstarch
2 tbsp cold water
non-iodized salt and pepper, to taste
½ cup slivered blanched almonds

1. Cut chicken in pieces to fit feed tube snugly. Freeze chicken until quite stiff, about 2 hours. You should be able to insert the point of a knife into the chicken.
2. Insert Slicer in food processor. Slice chicken, using firm pressure. (If

chicken isn't frozen firmly enough, it won't slice easily. If chicken is fully frozen, partially thaw it just until you can insert the point of a knife. If you don't have a processor, chicken can be thinly sliced on the diagonal using a chef's knife.)

3. Slicer: Stack mushrooms on their sides in the feed tube. Slice, using light pressure. Slice onion, using medium pressure.
4. Heat oil in a wok. (A large skillet may be used instead.) Add chicken pieces when oil is nearly smoking; stir-fry over high heat for 2 minutes, until chicken is white. Add mushrooms and stir-fry for 1 minute. Add onion, garlic, ginger, and peas and stir-fry 2 minutes longer.
5. Add chicken broth and sesame oil. Cover and let simmer for 2 minutes.
6. Dissolve cornstarch in cold water. Uncover wok and push chicken and vegetables up the sides. Stir cornstarch mixture into boiling liquid at the bottom of the wok. Cook just until thickened, stirring constantly. (If not thick enough, add 1 to 2 teaspoons cornstarch dissolved in a little water.)
7. Add seasonings and almonds and mix well. Serve immediately.

Yield: 4 servings. If frozen, vegetables won't be crispy.

Chicken and Rice Casserole

This one-dish meal is so easy, and it's perfect comfort food.

    1 cup long-grain rice
    2 onions, chopped
    2 cloves garlic, minced
    1 green pepper, chopped
    1 cup SALT-FREE tomato sauce or Fresh Tomato Sauce (see page 189)
    1 ¼ cups water
    3 lb chicken, cut up
    ¾ tsp non-iodized salt
    ¼ tsp pepper
    ⅛ tsp each dried basil and oregano

1. Combine rice, onions, garlic and green pepper in the bottom of a sprayed 2-quart oblong casserole. Add tomato sauce and water.
2. Arrange chicken skin-side down in a single layer on top of rice and vegetables. Sprinkle with seasonings.
3. Bake covered in a preheated 350ºF oven for 45 minutes. Turn chicken pieces over and bake covered 20 to 30 minutes longer, until tender.

Yield: 4 servings. Freezes and reheats very well.

Variation: *Omit tomato sauce and water. Replace with 2 ¼ cups SALT-FREE chicken broth. Sliced mushrooms make a delicious addition.*

Chicken Fingers

These are a favorite of kids of all ages!

> 4 boneless, skinless single chicken breasts, trimmed of fat (1 ½ lb)
> 1 cup matzo meal
> ¼ cup sesame seeds, optional
> non-iodized salt and pepper to taste
> ½ tsp paprika
> ½ tsp dried basil
> 2 egg whites
> oil for frying

1. Rinse chicken; pat dry. Cut each breast into strips about 1 inch wide. In a plastic bag, combine matzo meal, sesame seeds and seasonings. In a bowl, beat egg whites until frothy.
2. Dip chicken in egg white, then drop a few pieces at a time into matzo meal mixture. Shake to fully coat chicken.
3. Brown in hot oil over medium heat on both sides until crisp and golden, about 3 to 4 minutes per side. Do not crowd frying pan. Drain well on paper towels.

Yield: About 24 chicken fingers. These reheat and/or freeze well.

Serving Suggestions:

- *Kids love to dip chicken fingers (and their own fingers too) in honey! You can also serve these with Homemade LID-safe Ketchup (see recipe, page 183) or Super Salsa (see page 257).*
- *These are also delicious dipped in Pineapple Dipping Sauce or Sweet and Tangy Apricot Sauce (see pages 184 and 185).*

Cranberry Chicken Meatballs

2 lb minced chicken
1 onion, halved
1 carrot, peeled and cut in 1-inch chunks
1 stalk celery
2 egg whites
½ tsp garlic powder
1 ½ tsp non-iodized salt
¼ tsp pepper
⅓ cup matzo meal
2 – 14 oz cans SALT-FREE jellied cranberry sauce or Homemade Cranberry Sauce (see recipe, page 182)
½ tsp cinnamon
2 cups SALT-FREE tomato sauce or Fresh Tomato Sauce (see recipe, page 189)

1. If chicken isn't already minced, put about half of the chicken that you've cut in 1-inch chunks into the processor bowl, which has been fitted with the Steel Blade. Process until finely minced, about 10 seconds. Transfer to a mixing bowl. Repeat twice more with remaining chicken breasts, adding each in turn to the mixing bowl.
2. Process onion, carrot, and celery until minced. Add egg whites and

seasonings and process a few seconds longer. Add with matzo meal to minced chicken. Mix well.

3. Wet hands and form small meatballs as an appetizer or larger ones as a main course. Place on a foil-lined cookie sheet, which has been lightly greased. Bake uncovered at 350ºF for about 25 to 30 minutes.

4. Steel Blade: Place cranberry sauce and cinnamon in processor bowl. Add tomato sauce through feed tube while machine is running. Process until blended. Transfer to a large ovenproof casserole. Add meatballs and bake uncovered at 350ºF for 1 hour, basting occasionally. Serve on a bed of fluffy white rice.

Yield: 6 to 8 servings as a main course, 10 to 12 servings as an appetizer. May be frozen.

Cranberry Meatballs: *Substitute 2 lb lean ground beef or veal for the chicken.*

Doug's Quick Chicken Dinner

A complete meal for one or two in a single dish. Recipe doubles easily. My son Doug is an excellent chef. He loves boneless chicken in any form whatsoever. With his hearty appetite, Doug cooks and eats this whole meal by himself with absolutely no problem!

1 small onion, chopped
1 or 2 potatoes, peeled and cut into chunks
½ green pepper, sliced
1 carrot, peeled and sliced
½ stalk celery, sliced
2 single boneless, skinless chicken breasts (about ½ lb)
½ cup SALT-FREE tomato sauce or Fresh Tomato Sauce (see page 189)
non-iodized salt to taste
pepper, dried basil, and garlic powder to taste

1. Combine vegetables in a 1-quart microsafe casserole. Microwave covered on HIGH for 5 minutes, or until potatoes and carrots are almost tender. Stir halfway through and at end of cooking time.
2. Place chicken breasts over vegetables, with the thicker parts towards the outside of the casserole. Combine tomato sauce with seasonings and pour over chicken. (Sauce helps the chicken cook evenly.)
3. Microwave covered on HIGH for 4 to 5 minutes, until chicken is done, rotating the dish ¼ turn at half time. Let stand covered for 2 minutes.

Yield: 1 large or 2 moderate servings.

- *You can use any vegetables you like. Be sure to microwave them until almost tender before adding chicken breasts and sauce. This will ensure that the vegetables will be done but the chicken won't be overcooked.*
- *To double the recipe: Double all the ingredients, except use just ¾ cup of SALT-FREE sauce. Use a 2-quart microsafe casserole. Microwave vegetables covered on HIGH for 7 to 8 minutes, stirring at half time. Potatoes and carrots should be almost tender. Add chicken, sauce, and seasonings. Microwave covered on HIGH 7 to 8 minutes longer, until chicken is cooked, turning chicken over at half time. Let stand covered for 3 to 4 minutes before serving.*
- *SALT-FREE chicken broth can be used instead of SALT-FREE tomato sauce.*

Freeze with Ease Turkey Chili
(See recipe, page 114.)

Grilled Chicken Kabobs
These make a marvelous main dish for family or friends. Serve them at your next BBQ!

1. Prepare chicken as directed in the recipe for Mini Grilled Chicken Kabobs (see page 160), but cut into 2-inch chunks. (You should get 6 pieces from each breast.) Also cut 1 red onion into chunks. Alternately

thread chicken, peppers and onions onto 8-inch presoaked wooden skewers. Brush with some of the marinade.

2. Preheat BBQ or broiler. Grill or broil kabobs about 5 inches from the heat for about 8 to 10 minutes, turning skewers so chicken and vegetables will cook evenly. Do not overcook or chicken will be dry. Serve with Pineapple Dipping Sauce (see recipe, page 184).

Yield: 8 kabobs (4 servings). Do not freeze. Recipe can be doubled or tripled for a crowd.

Herb Roasted Chicken

So flavorful, so moist! This recipe will become part of your regular repertoire.

3 lb chicken, cut into pieces
2 to 3 cloves garlic, crushed
½ tsp each of dried basil, oregano, and rosemary
¼ tsp dried thyme
1 tsp Hungarian paprika
non-iodized salt to taste
freshly ground pepper
1 tbsp olive oil

1. Wash chicken well and pat dry. Loosen chicken skin but don't remove it. Rub flesh of chicken with garlic, seasonings, and olive oil. Cover chicken and marinate at least an hour (or preferably overnight) in the refrigerator to allow the flavor of the herbs to penetrate.

2. Preheat oven to 400°F. Place chicken pieces skin-side down on a rack in a greased foil-lined pan. Roast uncovered for 15 minutes. Reduce heat 350°F. Roast chicken skin-side up for 1 hour, or until golden and juices run clear. Baste occasionally. Remove skin before serving, if desired.

Yield: 6 servings. Recipe may be doubled or tripled, if desired. Freezes well.

Shortcut BBQ Chicken: *Prepare chicken as directed in Step 1. Preheat the BBQ or grill. Place chicken in a Pyrex casserole and microwave covered on HIGH for 8 to 9 minutes. Turn chicken pieces over, moving small pieces to the center. Microwave 7 to 8 minutes longer. Immediately transfer partly cooked chicken to hot BBQ. Cook 15 to 20 minutes longer, until crispy and golden. Remove skin before serving, if desired.*

Herb Roasted Chicken with Potatoes

4 lb chicken, cut up
non-iodized salt and ground pepper, to taste
1 tsp paprika (preferably Hungarian)
½ tsp dry mustard
½ tsp dried oregano
½ tsp dried basil
¼ tsp dried thyme
2 cloves garlic
1 large onion, quartered
½ cup SALT-FREE chicken broth or broth from Free Chicken Soup
(see recipe, page 83) or water
4 medium potatoes, peeled

1. Place chicken pieces in a large greased roasting pan and sprinkle with seasonings.
2. Insert Steel Blade in processor. Drop garlic through feed tube while machine is running. Process until minced. Scrape down sides of bowl. Add onion and process with 3 or 4 quick on/off turns, until coarsely chopped. Rub onion and garlic over chicken. If possible, let stand at least ½ hour to develop maximum flavor.
3. Add broth or water. Roast uncovered at 325ºF for about 2 hours, or until tender and golden.

4. About half an hour before chicken is done, insert Slicer in processor. Cut potatoes to fit feed tube. Slice, using firm pressure. Add potatoes to chicken and sprinkle with additional seasonings. Baste occasionally, adding extra liquid if necessary.

Yield: 4 to 6 servings. Chicken freezes well, but omit potatoes if you plan to freeze this dish. Recipe may be doubled.

Honey Crumb Chicken

This recipe for crumb-coated chicken from my friend Marilyn Goodman is delicious, yet so easy to prepare!

> 6 boneless, skinless single chicken breasts
> ⅓ cup honey
> 1 tbsp Homemade Low Iodine Mustard (see recipe below)
> non-iodized salt and ground pepper, to taste
> ½ tsp each of garlic powder and paprika
> ½ to ¾ cup matzo meal

1. Preheat oven to 375°F. Rinse chicken; remove excess fat. In a small bowl, combine honey with mustard; mix well. Coat chicken with honey-mustard mixture. Sprinkle on both sides with seasonings and crumbs.
2. Arrange chicken in a single layer in a sprayed oblong casserole. Bake uncovered at 375°F for 30 to 35 minutes, until golden, turning chicken over halfway through cooking.

Yield: 6 servings. Freezes well.

Homemade Low Iodine Mustard: *Blend ¼ cup dry mustard with 2 to 3 tbsp water. Store covered in the refrigerator for up to a month.*

Limelight Roast Chicken

Gloria Schachter of Montreal gave me this moist and luscious chicken recipe, which I've adapted. Yummy!

> 3 ½ lb whole chicken
> non-iodized salt and freshly ground pepper to taste
> 1 tsp dried basil
> 3 limes
> 1 or 2 stalks celery, cut into chunks
> ¼ cup chopped parsley or coriander (cilantro)

1. Rinse chicken and dry well. Loosen skin; rub seasonings inside the cavity and under skin of chicken. Squeeze juice of one lime over chicken. Marinate for one hour at room temperature, or cover and marinate in the fridge overnight.
2. Pierce limes with a fork. Place limes, celery, and parsley or coriander inside the chicken. Close up openings with metal skewers. Place chicken on its side in a roasting pan.
3. Preheat oven to 425ºF. Roast uncovered for 20 minutes. Turn chicken onto its other side and roast 20 minutes more. Reduce heat to 350ºF and roast breast-side up 20 minutes longer, until golden and crisp.
4. Remove chicken from oven. Strain fat from pan juices. Place pan juices in a gravy boat. Cut up chicken. Remove skin, limes, celery and parsley. Garnish with additional lime slices.

Yield: 6 servings. Reheats and/or freezes well. Recipe can be doubled for company.

Marinated Herb Chicken

Simply scrumptious!

3 lb chicken, cut up
1 clove garlic
½ cup olive or canola oil
2 tsp non-iodized salt
¼ tsp pepper
¼ tsp dried oregano
1 cup all-purpose flour
1 tsp paprika (preferably Hungarian)

1. Wash chicken pieces and dry well. Trim off excess fat. Place in a 9-inch by 13-inch baking dish.
2. Insert Steel Blade in processor. Drop garlic through feed tube while machine is running. Process until minced. Add oil, salt, pepper, and oregano. Process a few seconds to blend. Drizzle over chicken and marinate 3 to 4 hours (or overnight) in refrigerator. Turn once or twice for even marinating.
3. Place flour in plastic bag and add chicken pieces, one or two at a time. Shake to coat. Dip again in marinade. Arrange in a single layer on a sprayed foil-lined cookie sheet. Sprinkle with paprika. Bake uncovered at 425°F for 1 hour, until golden and crispy.

Yield: 4 servings. May be frozen.

Mini Grilled Chicken Kabobs

Mini kabobs make great appetizers. To serve this as a main dish, prepare Grilled Chicken Kabobs (see recipe, page 154).

4 boneless, skinless single chicken breasts, trimmed of fat
(about 1 ½ lb)
1 red and 1 green pepper
¼ cup olive oil
3 tbsp lemon juice
non-iodized salt and pepper, to taste
1 tsp fresh minced basil (or ½ tsp dried basil)
32 four-inch wooden skewers (soak in cold water for 20 minutes)
1 cup Pineapple Dipping Sauce (see page 184)

1. Rinse chicken and cut into 1-inch pieces. Pat dry with paper towels. (You should get about 8 to 10 pieces from each chicken breast.) Cut peppers into ½ inch chunks.
2. Blend olive oil with lemon juice, salt, pepper, and basil in a glass bowl. Add chicken and peppers; mix well. Marinate for at least ½ hour. (Can be prepared in advance and refrigerated up to 24 hours.)
3. Line a baking sheet with foil; spray with non-stick spray. Place a piece of chicken on each skewer. Put a piece of red pepper on one end and green pepper on the other end. (Kabobs can be assembled in advance. Refrigerate kabobs.
4. At serving time, bake at 400ºF for 10 to 12 minutes. (Kabobs can also be broiled or grilled for 3 or 4 minutes per side. Do not overcook.) Serve with Pineapple Dipping Sauce.

Yield: 32 miniature kabobs. Reheat at 400ºF for 6 to 8 minutes. Do not freeze.

Moo Goo Guy Pan

4 boneless, skinless single chicken breasts
½ tsp non-iodized salt
¼ tsp pepper
2 tsp cornstarch
1 green pepper, halved and seeded
2 cups mushrooms
2 tbsp canola or peanut oil
1 clove garlic, peeled and halved

1. Wash and dry chicken thoroughly. Cut into 1-inch squares with a sharp knife. Mix with salt, pepper, and cornstarch.
2. Insert Slicer in processor. Slice green pepper and mushrooms, using light pressure. Place on paper towels to absorb excess moisture.
3. Heat oil in a wok or deep skillet. Add garlic and brown for a minute or two. Discard garlic. Make sure oil is nearly smoking, then add chicken and stir constantly over high heat for 2 or 3 minutes, until pieces turn white. Push chicken up sides of wok.
4. Add mushrooms and green pepper and stir-fry for 2 minutes. Adjust seasonings to taste and mix to combine all ingredients.

Yield: 4 servings. Do not freeze, or vegetables will lose their crispness.

Variation: *One large onion, thinly sliced, may be added just before the mushrooms and green pepper in Step 4. Stir-fry onion for 1 minute. Add mushrooms and green pepper and continue with recipe.*

Pineapple Chicken

2 chickens, cut in eighths
non-iodized salt and pepper, to taste
1 tbsp paprika
2 cloves garlic
1 cup SALT-FREE canned tomato sauce or Fresh Tomato Sauce
(see recipe, page 189)
6 oz can frozen concentrated orange juice, slightly thawed
¼ cup honey
½ tsp dry mustard
½ tsp cinnamon
½ tsp ground ginger
14 oz can pineapple chunks
1 medium seedless orange

1. Sprinkle chicken with salt, pepper, and paprika on all sides. Place in a sprayed roasting pan.
2. Insert Steel Blade in processor. Drop garlic through feed tube while machine is running. Process until minced. Scrape down sides of bowl. Add tomato sauce, orange juice, honey, seasonings, and ½ cup juice from canned pineapple. (Reserve the rest of the pineapple juice in case you need it to baste the chicken.) Process for 2 or 3 seconds to blend. Pour over chicken.
3. Bake uncovered for about 2 hours at 350ºF. Baste occasionally. If sauce cooks down too much, add a little reserved pineapple juice. Add drained pineapple chunks 5 minutes before done.
4. Slicer: Cut orange in half lengthwise. Slice, using medium pressure. (You should have beautiful paper-thin slices of orange.) Serve chicken on a bed of fluffy white rice. Spoon sauce over chicken, garnish with orange slices.

Yield: 8 servings. Freezes well, but don't garnish until serving time.

Quick and Spicy Turkey Meat Loaf

So simple! This sauce is also great with chicken, burgers, or meatballs, or served over rice.

14 oz can SALT-FREE jellied cranberry sauce or Homemade Cranberry
Sauce (see recipe, page 182)
1 ¾ cups SALT-FREE bottled salsa or homemade Super Salsa (see
recipe, page 257)
3 tbsp white sugar or honey
1 tbsp lemon juice
non-iodized salt and ground pepper, to taste
1 lb lean ground turkey breast
⅓ cup matzo meal or quick-cooking oats

1. Preheat oven to 400°F. Melt cranberry sauce in a saucepan on medium heat (or microwave on HIGH for 3 minutes, until melted). Stir well. Mix in salsa, white sugar or honey, and lemon juice. Season with salt and pepper. Use half of sauce for this recipe. (Leftover sauce keeps for 10 days in the refrigerator or can be frozen.)
2. In a bowl, combine ground turkey with ½ cup of sauce, matzo meal or oats, salt, and pepper; mix lightly to blend. Shape into a loaf and place in a sprayed oblong casserole or loaf pan. Pour 1 cup of sauce over the top of the loaf. Bake uncovered at 400°F for 45 minutes.

Yield: 4 to 5 servings. Reheats and/or freezes well.

Variation: *Turkey mixture can be made into patties or mini-loaves. Baking time will be about 25 minutes.*

Saucy Chicken Livers

To complete this tasty meal, serve it on a bed of rice or LID-safe noodles.

1 lb chicken livers, halved
2 onions, quartered
1 green and 1 red pepper, halved and seeded
2 cups mushrooms
2 tbsp oil
1 cup fresh pea pods, ends trimmed
1 tbsp non-iodized salt
2 cloves garlic, crushed
1 to 2 tbsp honey, to taste
½ tsp ground ginger (or 1 tsp minced fresh ginger)
2 tbsp cornstarch, dissolved in ¼ cup cold water
1 tsp toasted sesame oil
freshly ground pepper

1. Broil chicken livers lightly on both sides. Set aside.
2. Insert Slicer into food processor. Slice onions, using medium pressure. Empty bowl and place onions on paper toweling to absorb excess moisture. Repeat with peppers, then mushrooms. Pat dry.
3. Heat oil in a large skillet or wok. Sauté onions for 1 to 2 minutes on medium-high heat, stirring. Remove from pan. Repeat with peppers, then with mushrooms.
4. Add pea pods to skillet along with sautéed vegetables and salt, garlic, honey, and ginger. Stir in chicken livers. Simmer for 2 or 3 minutes, stirring occasionally.
5. Make a well in the center and stir in cornstarch/water mixture and sesame oil. Cook until sauce is clear and thickened, about 2 minutes longer, stirring constantly. Add pepper to taste. Serve immediately.

Yield: 4 servings. Do not freeze, or vegetables will become soggy.

Variation: *Stir in ½ cup toasted slivered almonds or sprinkle with toasted sesame seeds.*

Sesame Baked Chicken

Instead of 4 boneless, skinless chicken breasts, substitute 3 lb chicken, cut in eighths, or 4 chicken breasts (with skin and bone). Proceed as directed for Sesame Fried Chicken (see below). Don't fry, but bake uncovered at 400ºF for 45 minutes to 1 hour, until done. This can be frozen, but it's preferable to underbake it slightly to avoid that "reheated" flavor.

Sesame Fried Chicken

¾ cup matzo meal
½ tsp non-iodized salt
dash of pepper
½ tsp paprika
¼ cup sesame seeds
2 egg whites plus 2 tbsp water
4 boneless, skinless single chicken breasts
3 tbsp canola oil, for frying

1. In a large plastic bag, combine matzo meal with seasonings and sesame seeds; mix well. In a pie plate, blend egg whites with water. Dip chicken pieces in beaten egg white, then in crumb mixture.
2. Heat oil in a large skillet. Brown chicken breasts on medium heat in hot oil about 5 minutes on each side, until golden and crispy. Drain on paper towels. May be reheated uncovered at 400ºF for 10 minutes on a cookie sheet.

Yield: 4 servings. May be frozen.

■ MEAT DISHES

Best Meatballs
These are delicious either as an appetizer or main dish. MMM-good!

Sauce:
9 oz jar all-natural, no-preservatives-added grape jelly
19 oz can SALT-FREE tomato juice
2 – 28 oz cans SALT-FREE tomatoes
½ cup honey
2 tbsp lemon juice
1 tsp non-iodized salt

Meatballs:
4 lb lean ground beef
1 cup matzo meal
4 egg whites
⅔ cup water
2 cloves garlic, minced
1 tbsp non-iodized salt
½ tsp pepper

1.   Combine sauce ingredients in a heavy-bottomed Dutch oven. Heat on low, stirring often to prevent jelly from scorching. Bring to simmering.
2.   Combine ground beef, matzo meal, egg whites, water, garlic, salt, and pepper in a large mixing bowl. Mix lightly to blend.
3.   Form small meatballs about the size of a walnut. Drop into simmering sauce and cook partially covered for 2 ½ to 3 hours, stirring occasionally. (Meatballs and sauce may also be baked covered in the oven at 325°F.)

Yield: About 100 meatballs. Freezes well. Tastes even better reheated.

Note: *Recipe may be halved, if desired. Veal may be substituted for the beef.*

Best-Ever Brisket

3 or 4 onions
4 to 5 lb brisket
2 tsp non-iodized salt
freshly ground pepper
1 tbsp paprika
1 tsp dry mustard
4 cloves garlic
⅓ cup apple juice
2 tbsp balsamic vinegar
2 to 3 tbsp honey or maple syrup

1. Insert Slicer in food processor. Cut onions to fit feed tube. Slice, using medium pressure. Place in the bottom of a large sprayed roasting pan. Rub brisket on all sides with salt, pepper, paprika, and mustard. Place in pan.
2. Steel Blade: Drop garlic through feed tube while machine is running. Process until minced. Add apple juice, balsamic vinegar, and honey or maple syrup; process 2 or 3 seconds longer. Pour mixture over brisket and rub into meat on all sides. Cover pan with aluminum foil. Let marinate at least 1 hour at room temperature, or overnight in the refrigerator.
3. Bake covered at 325°F. Allow 45 minutes per pound, or until meat is fork tender. Uncover for the last hour and baste occasionally. Let stand for 20 to 30 minutes before slicing. Reheat for a few minutes in pan gravy.

Yield: 8 to 10 servings. Freezes well. May be prepared a day or two in advance and refrigerated. Discard the hardened fat, then slice the brisket to desired thickness. Mouthwatering!

Braised Meatballs

So tasty, so easy! Adding club soda to the ground meat mixture produces a very light texture. Julia Feldman was kind enough to share her secret with me, and now I share it with you.

2 large onions, chopped
2 tbsp canola oil
1 lb ground beef or veal
2 egg whites
2 tbsp cream of wheat or matzo meal
2 tbsp club soda
¾ tsp non-iodized salt
¼ tsp pepper
½ tsp garlic powder
¾ cup water
1 tbsp honey
¾ to 1 tsp Hungarian paprika (to taste)

1. In a large skillet, sauté onions in hot oil on medium heat until golden, about 7 to 8 minutes.
2. Meanwhile, combine ground meat, egg whites, cream of wheat or matzo meal, club soda, salt, pepper, and garlic powder in a mixing bowl. Mix lightly to blend.
3. Add water and honey to skillet. Form meat mixture into small meatballs. (Wet your hands for easier shaping.) Add meatballs to skillet. Sprinkle with paprika.
4. Cover and simmer for 2 hours, adding more water if needed. Stir occasionally.

Yield: 3 to 4 servings. Freezes and/or reheats well. Serve with rice or potatoes and a salad.

Variation: *Add 2 cups frozen SALT-FREE California-style mixed vegetables (broccoli, cauliflower, carrots, green beans, and red peppers) in the last 5 minutes of cooking.*

Cabbage Rolls
(See recipe, page 110.)

Coca Cola Brisket

5 to 6 lb shelled beef brisket
2 or 3 cloves garlic
1 small onion, halved
2 tbsp vinegar or lemon juice
¼ cup apple or cranberry juice
1 tbsp lemon juice
½ cup oil
¼ cup honey
¼ cup Coca Cola
3 tbsp Homemade Low Iodine Ketchup (see recipe, page 183) OR 3 tbsp SALT-FREE tomato paste (to which you can add ½ tsp non-iodized salt)
1 tbsp non-iodized salt
ground pepper (about ¼ tsp)
1 tsp paprika

1. Place brisket in a large sprayed roasting pan.
2. Insert Steel Blade in food processor. Process garlic and onion until minced. Add remaining ingredients and process a few seconds longer to blend. Pour over brisket, making sure to cover all surfaces. Let marinate at room temperature for 1 to 2 hours, or overnight in the refrigerator. Cover roasting pan well with foil.

3. Cook at 300°F for 5 hours, until very tender (about 1 hour per pound). When cool, refrigerate. This will slice better the next day. Remove the hardened fat and discard.

Yield: 10 to 12 servings. Freezes and/or reheats well.

Grilled London Broil

Pretty as a picture—just take a look at the cover photo!

1 flank steak (1 ½ lb)
¼ cup balsamic vinegar
2 tbsp olive oil
1 tbsp orange juice
3 cloves minced garlic
1 tbsp honey
½ tsp non-iodized salt (or to taste)
freshly ground black pepper
1 tbsp minced fresh basil
dash of cayenne
Quick and Easy Tomato Sauce (see page 192)
Roasted Red Peppers, for garnish (see page 259)
additional basil leaves, for garnish

1. Place flank steak in a 9- by 13-inch glass baking dish.
2. Combine balsamic vinegar, olive oil, orange juice, garlic, honey, salt, pepper, basil, and cayenne in a glass measuring cup or bowl; mix well. Pour mixture evenly over and around the meat. Cover and marinate for 1 to 2 hours in the refrigerator. (Can be prepared in advance and marinated for up to 24 hours. Turn meat over once or twice during marinating.)
3. Prepare tomato sauce and set aside. (Can be prepared in advance and reheated.)

4. Heat the grill or broiler. Remove meat from marinade and pat dry. Discard marinade. Grill or broil meat about 4 to 5 minutes per side for medium rare, or until desired doneness. Remove from heat and let stand about 5 minutes for easier slicing.

5. To serve, cut diagonally across the grain into slices. Pour a thin layer of hot tomato sauce on each plate. Top with sliced steak. Garnish with roasted peppers and basil. Serve immediately.

Yield: 4 servings. Delicious hot or cold. Leftover steak can also be served on a bed of chilled greens.

TIPS AND SUBSTITUTIONS FOR MEAT-LOVERS ON A LID

- Soy sauce is not allowed in LID-safe recipes, so sprinkle a little onion powder or garlic powder on foods to give them a lift. Add a dash of curry powder, red pepper flakes, chili powder, or cayenne pepper to marinades, stir-fry dishes, and sauces.
- If a recipe calls for ¼ cup white wine, substitute 3 tbsp apple or orange juice, plus 1 tbsp lemon juice or rice vinegar for a flavor boost.
- If a recipe calls for ¼ cup red wine, substitute 3 tbsp cola beverage plus 1 tbsp balsamic vinegar.
- Always avoid cooking wines, as they're made with 1.5 % salt (to render them non-drinkable).

Marinated Roast

4 lb boneless chuck roast
2 to 3 cloves garlic
¼ cup oil
½ cup orange juice
½ cup apple juice

1 tbsp honey
½ tsp ground ginger
1 large or 2 medium onions, halved
1 red pepper, halved and seeded

1. Pierce roast deeply on both sides with a fork and place in a 9- by 13-inch Pyrex dish or roasting pan.
2. Insert Steel Blade in food processor. Drop garlic through feed tube while machine is running. Process until minced. Add remaining ingredients except onion and process for a few seconds to blend. Pour over meat. Cover and marinate in refrigerator overnight, turning meat once. (Meat may also be marinated at room temperature for 1 hour.)
3. Slicer: Slice onion and red pepper, using medium pressure. (This may be done at the same time you prepare the marinade, while the processor bowl is already in use, to save cleanup the next day. Store sliced onion and peppers in a plastic bag in the refrigerator.)
4. Drain most of the marinade from the meat. Refrigerate marinade until just before serving time. Add onion and peppers to meat, cover tightly and bake at 325ºF for about 3 hours, or until tender. Let stand 20 minutes before slicing.
5. Heat reserved marinade in a saucepan and serve over slices of roast.

Yield: 8 servings. May be frozen. Delicious with rice and steamed broccoli.

Old-Fashioned Hamburgers
(See recipe, page 115.)

Oven-Roasted Short Ribs

3 cloves garlic
6 to 8 strips short ribs (flanken)
non-iodized salt, to taste
pepper and paprika, to taste
½ tsp dried basil
½ tsp dried oregano
¼ tsp dried dill weed
3 onions, halved
½ cup water, apple juice or SALT-FREE tomato juice
1 tbsp balsamic vinegar
1 tsp white sugar

1. Insert Steel Blade in processor. Drop garlic through feed tube while machine is running, Process until minced. Remove from processor bowl with a rubber spatula and spread over meat. Add seasonings and rub into meat on all sides. Place in a large roaster.
2. Slicer: Slice onions, using medium pressure. Add to roasting pan. Combine water, apple, or tomato juice with balsamic vinegar and sugar; add to pan.
3. Cover and bake at 325°F for 2 hours. Uncover and cook 1 hour longer, basting occasionally. Sliced potatoes may be added the last ½ hour, if desired.

Yield: 4 to 6 servings. May be frozen, but omit potatoes.

Red Hot Chili

Cocoa gives a rich, dark color to this chili. If there's an excuse to put chocolate into a recipe, I'll find it!

> 1 ½ lb lean ground beef
> 2 cloves garlic
> 2 large onions, quartered
> 1 green pepper, cut in chunks
> 2 ½ cups SALT-FREE tomato sauce
> 5 ½ oz can SALT-FREE tomato paste plus ½ can water
> 19 oz can SALT-FREE red kidney beans, drained (or 2 cups cooked kidney beans)
> 1 to 2 tbsp chili powder (to taste)
> 1 tbsp unsweetened pure cocoa powder (LID-safe)
> 1 tsp non-iodized salt
> ½ tsp pepper
> ½ tsp cumin
> red pepper flakes, if desired

1. Preheat a large Dutch oven and add ground beef. Break up with a spoon.
2. Insert Steel Blade in processor. Drop garlic through feed tube and process until minced. Process onions and green pepper with quick on/off turns, until finely chopped. Add to Dutch oven. Brown meat and vegetables over medium-high heat, stirring often.
3. Add remaining ingredients. Reduce heat and simmer uncovered for about 1 hour, stirring often. Adjust seasonings to taste.

Yield: 4 to 6 servings. Even better the next day. Freezes well. Serve over LID-safe noodles or rice, or in a bowl with LID-safe flatbread and chopped onions.

Stuffed Peppers

(See recipe, page 119.)

Super Stew

Cooking time in the microwave is less than half of conventional cooking time. Besides, microwaved stew never sticks to the pot. Also, check out the effortless oven-baked version.

3 cloves garlic, minced
2 onions, chopped
2 stalks celery, chopped
2 tbsp oil
2 lb stewing beef or veal, cut in 1 inch cubes
4 carrots, peeled, trimmed, and cut in 1 inch chunks
4 medium potatoes, peeled and cut in 1 inch chunks
5 ½ oz can SALT-FREE tomato paste
½ cup apple juice
1 tbsp balsamic vinegar
1 cup SALT-FREE chicken broth or broth from Free Chicken Soup
(see recipe, page 83)
1 tsp non-iodized salt
freshly ground pepper
1 tsp dried basil
¼ tsp dried thyme

1. Combine garlic, onions and celery with oil in a deep 3- or 4-quart microsafe casserole. Microwave uncovered on HIGH for 3 to 4 minutes. Add meat; microwave uncovered on HIGH for 5 to 6 minutes. Stir, moving less cooked portions towards the outside of the casserole. Microwave on HIGH for 4 to 6 minutes longer, until meat is no longer pink.
2. Add remaining ingredients; mix well. Cover with casserole lid. Microwave covered on HIGH for 15 minutes, until bubbling. Mix well.

3. If casserole is very deep, place a sheet of waxed paper or cooking parchment on surface of stew to trap the steam. Cover with casserole lid. Reduce power to MEDIUM (50%) and microwave 1 hour and 20 minutes longer, stirring 2 or 3 times. Meat should be covered by sauce to prevent it from turning dark. Let stand covered for 15 to 30 minutes (or longer if you have the time). Flavor improves with standing.

Yield: 4 to 6 servings. Freezes well, but omit potatoes.

- *After cooking, stew can be chilled. Excess fat will congeal and can be removed easily. Stew tastes even better the next day.*
- *If desired, omit potatoes. Total cooking time for stew will be reduced by about 10 minutes. Serve stew and its luscious sauce over oodles of LID-safe noodles or rice. So good!*

Variation: *To bake stew in the oven, in Step 1, combine all ingredients except potatoes in a large ovenproof casserole. Bake covered in a preheated 325ºF oven for 2 ½ hours. Add potatoes and bake covered for 45 to 60 minutes longer, until meat and potatoes are tender.*

Sweet and Sour Brisket

The brisket is partially cooked, then sliced and returned to the gravy to finish cooking and absorb the delicious pan juices.

2 medium onions, chopped
3 ½ to 4 lb brisket
2 tsp non-iodized salt
freshly ground pepper
1 tsp dried oregano
2 cloves garlic, minced
1 cup SALT-FREE tomato sauce or Fresh Tomato Sauce (see recipe, page 189)

⅓ to ½ cup maple syrup or honey (to taste)
⅓ to ½ cup wine vinegar (to taste)

1. Place onions in the bottom of a large roasting pan that has been sprayed with cooking spray. Rub brisket with seasonings. Place in roasting pan. Combine remaining ingredients and add to roasting pan. (Can be prepared in advance, covered and refrigerated overnight.)
2. Preheat oven to 325ºF. Cook brisket covered, about 2 hours. (Allow 30 minutes per pound.)
3. Remove brisket from oven and let stand covered for 20 to 30 minutes. Slice across the grain.
4. Place brisket slices back into the sauce. Cover and bake 1 hour longer, until tender, basting occasionally.

Yield: 8 servings. Freezes and/or reheats well.

Veal Cacciatore

2 lb veal cutlets, pounded thin
non-iodized salt and pepper, to taste
3 large cloves garlic
¼ cup fresh parsley (or 1 tbsp dried)
2 onions, cut in chunks
19 oz can SALT-FREE tomatoes (or 5 to 6 fresh tomatoes)
5 ½ oz can SALT-FREE tomato paste
½ tsp dried basil
½ tsp dried oregano
1 tsp white sugar
¾ tsp non-iodized salt
¼ tsp pepper
1 tbsp oil
1 bay leaf

3 tbsp orange or apple juice
1 tbsp lemon juice or balsamic vinegar

1. Sprinkle veal lightly on both sides with salt and pepper. Set aside.
2. Insert Steel Blade in processor. Drop garlic through feed tube while machine is running. Process until minced. (It's not necessary to peel the garlic as it will dissolve during cooking.) Add parsley and onions. Process until minced. Empty into a large sprayed roasting pan.
3. Process half the canned (or fresh) tomatoes and half the tomato paste with the remaining ingredients until blended. Add to roasting pan. Repeat with remaining tomatoes and tomato paste. Add to roasting pan and stir to blend. Place veal cutlets in casserole; spoon the sauce over veal.
4. Cover tightly and bake at 325ºF for 1 hour. Uncover and bake ½ hour longer, or until meat is tender.

Yield: 4 to 6 servings. Freezes well.

Note: *If desired, add 2 green peppers and 2 cups of mushrooms. Slice on the Slicer, using light pressure. Sauté briefly in 2 tbsp oil. Garnish veal at serving time. Delicious with LID-safe spaghetti or rice. I've also made this dish using veal chops, and it's equally delicious. If using veal chops, the total cooking time will be 2 hours.*

Veal Normande

This delicious veal dish can be made either in the microwave or on top of the stove.

2 cloves garlic, minced
1 onion, chopped
1 green pepper, chopped
1 tbsp oil
2 lb lean stewing veal, cut in 1-inch pieces
¾ tsp non-iodized salt

freshly ground pepper

½ tsp dried rosemary or tarragon

1 tbsp chopped parsley

¾ cup SALT-FREE chicken broth

⅓ cup apple juice

1 tbsp lemon juice

5 ½ oz can SALT-FREE tomato paste

1. Combine garlic, onion, green pepper and oil in a shallow 2-quart microsafe casserole. Microwave uncovered on HIGH for 5 minutes, until tender.

2. Add remaining ingredients and mix well. Make sure that meat is completely submerged in the liquid. Cover with casserole lid or parchment paper. Microwave covered on HIGH for 10 minutes, or until bubbling. Stir well.

3. Microwave covered on MEDIUM (50%) for 1 hour, stirring twice. Meat should be fairly tender.

4. Let stand covered for at least 15 minutes. (It's even tastier and more tender if prepared in advance and reheated.) Serve with LID-safe noodles or rice and green peas.

Yield: 4 to 6 servings. Freezes and/or reheats well.

1. **Conventional Method:** Coat veal with 2 tbsp flour seasoned with non-iodized salt, pepper, and paprika. Heat 2 tbsp oil in a large skillet. Add veal and brown on medium heat on all sides. Remove veal from pan and set aside. In the same skillet, sauté onion, garlic, and green pepper in 1 tbsp oil for 5 to 7 minutes, until tender. Add veal to skillet along with remaining ingredients. (You can also add 1 cup of SALT-FREE tomato sauce.) Cover and simmer until meat is tender, about 1 ½ to 2 hours.

Zelda's Meat Loaf

This should really be called "Used to be Zelda's Meat Loaf" Marty Kaplan gave me his mother's recipe, which was a lot of work to prepare and fairly high in calories. I used my processor to speed up the preparation time, and adapted the recipe for the new millennium. Zelda didn't stuff and roll her meat loaf, but I do. It makes a pretty pinwheel effect when sliced.

2 lb ground turkey (see tips)
1 onion
1 cup mushrooms
½ of a green pepper
2 fresh tomatoes
1 potato, peeled
1 large carrot
1 or 2 cloves garlic, crushed
½ cup SALT-FREE chicken broth or broth from Free Chicken Soup (see recipe, page 83) or water
1 tsp non-iodized salt
¼ tsp pepper
¼ tsp dried basil
¼ tsp dried thyme
¼ to ⅓ cup matzo meal or quick-cooking oats
½ cup sun-dried tomatoes, cut into strips (see tips)
½ to ¾ cup SALT-FREE tomato sauce (see tips) or Quick and Easy Tomato Sauce (see recipe, page 192)

1. Preheat oven to 375°F. Place ground turkey in a large mixing bowl.
2. In the processor using the Steel Blade, chop onion, mushrooms and green pepper, using quick on/offs. Place vegetables in a microsafe bowl and microwave on HIGH for 5 minutes, until tender.

3. Meanwhile, chop fresh tomatoes in the processor and add to ground turkey. Finely mince potato, carrot, and garlic on the Steel Blade. Add to turkey along with chicken broth or water, seasonings, and matzo meal or oats. Add the microwaved vegetables and mix lightly to blend.
4. Place meat mixture on a large sheet of plastic wrap and pat it into a rectangle about ½ inch thick. Place sun-dried tomatoes in 3 or 4 rows crosswise on the rectangle. Roll up the meat like a jelly roll. Discard plastic wrap.
5. Transfer meat loaf to a sprayed loaf pan and drizzle tomato sauce over the top. Bake uncovered at 375ºF about 1 hour. Add a little extra sauce before the end of cooking if the top gets too dry. Drain off any excess fat, slice and serve.

Yield: 8 servings. Reheats and/or freezes well. Delicious with baked or mashed potatoes and steamed green beans.

Tips:
*   *You can substitute extra-lean ground beef or half beef and half veal. Minced chicken breast can also be used.*
*   *If using oil-packed sun-dried tomatoes, rinse well to remove excess oil; pat dry. You can substitute steamed asparagus or strips of Roasted Red Peppers (see recipe, page 259) if you like.*
*   *To keep turkey meat loaf moist during cooking, I top it with a little sauce, but if using ground beef instead, adding the sauce is a matter of personal preference.*

■ MARINADES AND SAUCES

Chinese Sweet and Sour Sauce

Delicious with chicken, or as a dipping sauce with LID dumplings as a snack.

½ cup Homemade Low Iodine Ketchup (see recipe, page 183)
½ cup vinegar
¾ cup water
3 tbsp lemon juice
1 ¼ cups white sugar
½ cup honey (or to taste)
¼ cup cornstarch dissolved in ¼ cup cold water

1.   Combine Homemade Low Iodine Ketchup, vinegar, ¾ cup water, lemon juice, sugar, and honey in an 8-cup Pyrex measure and stir well. Microwave uncovered on HIGH for 6 to 7 minutes, until boiling, stirring at half time.
2.   Stir cornstarch mixture into sauce. Microwave on HIGH 2 minutes longer, until bubbling and thickened.

Yield: 3 cups sauce. Sauce will keep about 1 month in the refrigerator.

Cranberry Sauce

For garnish with meat, vegetables, or anything you like.

12 oz fresh or frozen cranberries
1 ¼ cups white sugar
½ cup water or orange juice
1 tsp grated orange rind

1.   Combine all ingredients in a 3-quart microsafe casserole. Mix well; cover with parchment paper or casserole lid. Microwave covered on HIGH for

5 minutes. Stir well. Cover and microwave 5 to 7 minutes longer, until cranberries pop and sauce has thickened. Let stand covered until cool. Transfer to a serving bowl and chill for 3 to 4 hours.

Yield: About 2 cups. Freezes well. This will keep for several weeks in the refrigerator if kept in a tightly sealed container.

Homemade Low Iodine Ketchup
This delicious ketchup takes moments to make in a blender or food processor and can be doubled easily.

½ small onion
1 or 2 cloves garlic
1 can (5 ½ oz) SALT-FREE tomato paste
⅔ cup white vinegar
3 tbsp water
⅓ cup white sugar
⅛ tsp pepper
⅛ tsp ground cloves
⅛ tsp cayenne

1.   Process onion and garlic in a food processor or blender until minced. Add remaining ingredients and process 10 to 15 seconds longer, until blended. If too thick, add a few drops of water.
2.   Transfer to a jar and store covered in the refrigerator for up to 3 weeks. Stir before using.

Yield: 1 ½ cups. Freezes well.

Variations: *Apple cider vinegar can be used instead of white vinegar. If desired, add ¼ tsp Italian seasoning (or a combination of dried basil and oregano).*

Pineapple Dipping Sauce

Delicious as a dipping sauce for chicken fingers, wings, or shish kabobs. Serve the extra sauce over rice.

 1 tbsp cornstarch
 3 tbsp cold water
 2 cups pineapple juice
 1 tbsp rice vinegar or lemon juice
 ⅓ cup minced red or green peppers
 ⅛ tsp red pepper flakes
 1 cup finely chopped pineapple (fresh or canned)
 2 green onions, minced
 1 tsp minced fresh ginger

1.	Blend cornstarch with cold water in a small bowl until smooth. Combine pineapple juice, vinegar or lemon juice, minced peppers, and red pepper flakes in a saucepan. Bring to a boil.
2.	Add cornstarch mixture and whisk over medium heat until thickened and smooth, about 2 to 3 minutes. Remove from heat and cool. Stir in pineapple, green onions and ginger.

Yield: About 3 cups. Sauce will keep about 4 to 5 days in the refrigerator, in a tightly closed container. You can make half the recipe, but it's so good, why bother?

Plum Sauce

Follow recipe for Chinese Sweet and Sour Sauce (see recipe, page 182) but substitute SALT-FREE canned pumpkin for the ketchup. (A few brands of canned pumpkin contain pure pumpkin without added salt.)

Sweet and Tangy Apricot Sauce or Glaze

2 cloves garlic, minced

½ small onion, minced

3 tbsp Homemade Low Iodine Ketchup (see recipe, page 183) or 1 tbsp SALT-FREE tomato paste (to which you can add a dash of non-iodized salt)

1 tbsp lemon or lime juice

½ cup apricot preserves

¼ cup orange marmalade

½ tsp non-iodized salt

½ tsp dry mustard

¼ tsp each ground ginger, chili powder, dried basil, and pepper

1. Combine all ingredients in a saucepan. Bring to a boil over medium heat. Boil for 30 to 45 seconds. (Or microwave on HIGH for 45 to 60 seconds, until bubbling.) Stir well to blend.

Yield: 1 cup sauce. Recipe may be doubled successfully. Sauce can be stored in a glass jar in the refrigerator for about 1 month. Delicious as either a glaze or dipping sauce for spare ribs, chicken wings, or chicken fingers. To prevent burning when using it as a glaze, don't brush it on until the last few minutes of cooking.

Yolk-Free Mayonnaise

No yolking! This is very easy to make and tastes delicious. Using pasteurized egg whites ensures food safety.

3 tbsp pasteurized liquid egg whites, thawed

2 tsp lemon juice

1 tsp dry mustard

¼ tsp non-iodized salt
freshly ground pepper
dash of cayenne
1 cup canola oil

1.   In a food processor fitted with the Steel Blade, combine egg whites, lemon juice, mustard, salt, pepper and cayenne. Process for 5 seconds to blend. While machine is running, add oil in a very slow, steady stream through the feed tube; process until thickened. Total time is approximately 45 seconds. Transfer to a clean container, cover, and refrigerate immediately.

Yield: About 1 cup. Keeps approximately 1 week. Do not freeze.

Serving Ideas:
- *This makes an excellent addition to chopped egg whites (discard the yolks) or diced cooked chicken for sandwiches and salads. Use in homemade potato salad along with Hard-Cooked Egg Whites (see page 60).*
- *Use this tasty yolk-free mayonnaise as a spread for LID-safe breads when making sandwiches.*
- **Veggie Dip:** *Add minced garlic, onion, chopped peppers, and your favorite herbs (e.g., basil, oregano, thyme, dill).*
- **Thousand Island Dressing:** *Combine ½ cup mayonnaise, ¼ cup Homemade Low Iodine Ketchup (see page 183), and ¼ cup minced onion. Season to taste.*

■ PASTA AND SAUCES

Cheater's High-Fiber Pasta Sauce

1 cup cooked lentils (or canned SALT-FREE lentils, well-drained)
1 jar SALT-FREE spaghetti sauce or 3 cups Quick and Easy Tomato Sauce (see recipe, page 192)
¼ cup water

1. Process lentils in your food processor using the Steel Blade until puréed. Add spaghetti sauce and process until well mixed, scraping down sides of bowl as needed.
2. Combine puréed mixture with water in a large saucepan. Bring to a boil and simmer partially covered for 10 minutes (or microwave uncovered on HIGH for 10 minutes), stirring occasionally.

Yield: About 4 cups. Freezes and/or reheats well.

Time Saving Secrets:
- *If using this sauce in dishes that require further cooking, don't bother precooking the sauce.*
- *To use sauce over spaghetti, simmer the sauce while pasta is cooking. If desired, stir some SALT-FREE frozen mixed vegetables into the sauce for extra nutrients. They'll defrost and cook with the sauce.*
- *If you have time, sauté some onions, peppers, mushrooms, and/or zucchini in a little olive oil. Combine veggies with sauce ingredients and simmer uncovered for 10 minutes.*

Chicken Primavera

There's a fair amount of preparation for this dish, but the results are worth it! Use your food processor to help you get the vegetables ready quickly. Vary the vegetables, if you wish. Good enough to serve to company!

4 boneless, skinless single chicken breasts (about 1 ½ lb)
2 tbsp olive or canola oil
non-iodized salt and pepper to taste
dried basil and oregano to taste
2 to 3 cloves garlic, minced
1 medium onion, sliced
½ green pepper, sliced
½ red pepper, sliced

1 cup mushrooms, sliced
1 cup broccoli florets
1 carrot, peeled and sliced
1 cup snow peas, if desired
2 cups Quick and Easy Tomato Sauce (see recipe, page 192)

1. Cut chicken into narrow strips. Place chicken and 1 tbsp oil in a 2-quart
    oval or rectangular microsafe casserole. Microwave uncovered on HIGH
    for 5 to 6 minutes, stirring every 2 minutes, until chicken is no longer
    pink. Sprinkle with seasonings. Cover to keep warm while microwaving
    remaining ingredients.
2. Combine garlic, onion and peppers with 1 tbsp oil in a 1-quart micro-
    safe bowl. Microwave uncovered on HIGH for 3 minutes. Stir in mush-
    rooms. Microwave on HIGH for 2 minutes longer, until tender-crisp.
    Drain; add to chicken.
3. Place broccoli and carrots in a microsafe casserole. Rinse with cold water;
    drain, but don't dry. Microwave covered on HIGH for 2 to 2 ½ minutes,
    until tender-crisp. Drain; add to chicken.
4. Remove tails from snow peas. Rinse and drain, but don't dry. Place in
    microsafe casserole. Microwave covered on HIGH for 1 minute, until
    tender-crisp. Add to chicken. Stir in tomato sauce. Season to taste. (Can
    be prepared up to this point.)
5. Microwave uncovered on HIGH for 4 to 6 minutes, or until heated
    through, stirring once or twice. (If refrigerated, increase time to 6 to 8
    minutes.) Delicious over LID-safe spaghetti, fettuccine, or rice.

Yield: 4 to 6 servings. If frozen, vegetables won't be as crisp.

Fresh Tomato Sauce

This is a wonderful recipe to make when the garden is overflowing with its harvest! The processor makes quick work of the vegetable preparation.

    2 cloves garlic
    2 onions
    1 stalk celery
    1 green pepper
    2 tbsp olive or canola oil
    4 lb ripe tomatoes, peeled and seeded (see method on page 107)
    5 ½ oz can SALT-FREE tomato paste
    1 tsp dried basil
    1 tsp dried oregano
    1 tbsp white sugar
    2 tsp non-iodized salt (or to taste)
    ¼ tsp pepper

1. Steel Blade: Drop garlic through feed tube while machine is running. Process until minced. Cut onions, celery, and green pepper in chunks. Process with several quick on/off turns, until coarsely chopped. Place vegetables in a 3-quart microsafe casserole along with oil. Microwave uncovered on HIGH for 5 minutes, until tender, stirring once.

2. Peel and seed tomatoes as directed on page 107. Process in batches on the Steel Blade using on/off turns, until coarsely chopped. Add to casserole along with remaining ingredients. Microwave covered on HIGH for 30 to 35 minutes, until slightly thickened and vegetables are tender, stirring occasionally

Yield: About 1 ½ quarts (6 cups) sauce. Sauce keeps about 10 days in the refrigerator. Freezes well.

Variation: *Add 1 tbsp Homemade Pesto (see recipe, page 191) to each cup of cooked sauce. Delicious over spaghetti, linguini, fettuccine, etc.*

High-Fiber Vegetarian Pasta Sauce

Adding mashed kidney beans or lentils to the sauce will thicken it, as well as increase the fiber content. No one will know! This is an excellent sauce to serve over spiral pasta such as fusilli or rotini. I also love to use it as a sauce for chicken breasts.

1 tbsp olive or vegetable oil
1 large onion, chopped
1 green pepper, chopped
1 red pepper, chopped
4 cloves garlic, crushed
3 medium zucchini, chopped (1 lb)
2 cups mushrooms, sliced
4 large fresh tomatoes, roughly chopped
2 cans (5 ½ oz each) SALT-FREE tomato paste
2 ½ cups water
non-iodized salt, to taste
½ tsp ground pepper
1 tsp dried basil
1 tsp white sugar
19 oz can SALT-FREE red kidney beans or lentils, rinsed, drained, and mashed (or 2 cups cooked kidney beans or lentils, mashed, see Note)

1. Conventional Method: Heat oil in a large, heavy-bottomed pot. Sauté onions and peppers for 4 minutes on medium heat. Add garlic, zucchini, and mushrooms and sauté 5 minutes longer. Add tomatoes and cook 3 minutes more. Add remaining ingredients and mix well. Bring to a boil. Simmer partly covered for 20 to 25 minutes, stirring occasionally.
2. Microwave Method: Combine oil, onions and peppers in a 3-quart microsafe casserole. Microwave covered on HIGH for 3 minutes.

Add garlic, zucchini, and mushrooms. Microwave 3 minutes more. Add tomatoes and microwave 3 minutes. Stir in remaining ingredients. Cover and microwave on HIGH for 20 minutes, stirring once or twice.

Yield: About 8 cups (8 servings). Freezes well.

Note: *If you have trouble digesting legumes, just omit them. Instead, thicken the sauce with oats, a super source of soluble fiber. Stir ⅓ cup of quick-cooking oats into sauce during the last 5 minutes of cooking.*

Optional: *If desired, purée all or part of the cooked sauce in batches in the food processor.*

Homemade Pesto

    2 cups tightly packed fresh basil leaves
    ½ cup fresh parsley
    4 large cloves garlic, peeled
    ¼ cup unsalted pine nuts
    ½ cup extra-virgin olive oil
    ½ tsp non-iodized salt
    freshly ground black pepper, to taste

1.   Wash basil and parsley; dry thoroughly. Start the processor and drop garlic through feed tube. Process until minced. Add nuts, basil, and parsley. Process until fine, about 15 seconds. Drizzle oil through feed tube while the machine is running. Process until blended. Season to taste.

Yield: About 1 cup. Store pesto in a glass jar in the refrigerator. It will keep up to 2 months if covered with a thin layer of oil. Freezes well.

Tips and Variations:
- *Use a combination of fresh basil and fresh spinach when basil is expensive. It works perfectly.*
- *Freeze basil in ice cube trays, then transfer the basil cubes to a freezer storage bag. Each cube contains about 2 tbsp basil. Use in sauces, salad dressings, or toss with LID-safe pasta or rice. Yummy!*

LID-Safe Homemade Pasta
(See recipe, page 103.)

Noodle Bake
(See recipe, page 104.)

Quick and Easy Tomato Sauce (Vegetarian Spaghetti Sauce)

This is an excellent, versatile, low-fat sauce that can be used in any recipe calling for tomato sauce (store-bought or homemade), marinara, or pasta sauce. It's wonderful with chicken, beans, and stews or as an ingredient in casseroles. I love to serve it with Grilled London Broil (see cover photo).

28 oz can SALT-FREE tomatoes (stewed, whole, or crushed)
5 ½ oz can SALT-FREE tomato paste
1 tbsp olive oil (preferably extra-virgin)
3 cloves garlic, crushed
non-iodized salt and pepper, to taste
¼ tsp cayenne or red pepper flakes
½ tsp dried oregano
1 to 2 tbsp fresh basil, minced (or ½ tsp dried)
½ tsp white sugar

1. Combine all ingredients in a large saucepan or covered microsafe casserole, breaking up tomatoes if necessary. To microwave, cook covered on HIGH for 10 minutes, stirring at half time. To cook conventionally, bring sauce to a boil, reduce heat and simmer covered for 20 to 25 minutes, stirring occasionally. Adjust seasonings to taste.

Yield: Approximately 4 cups sauce. Reheats and/or freezes well (see Note below.)

Note: *Freeze sauce in 1 cup portions for convenience, leaving about a half-inch space at the top of the container to allow for expansion. When you need some sauce, place the frozen container under running water briefly. Pop out the contents and transfer them to a microsafe bowl. Thaw on HIGH power (DEFROST takes too long). Stir several times. One cup of sauce takes about 5 minutes to thaw and reheat.*

Quicky Chicky with Fettuccine

This recipe takes about 20 minutes from start to finish. So easy, so good (and it's light in the calorie department too)! Boil the water for the pasta while chicken is cooking in the microwave.

> 1 large onion, cut in chunks
> 1 clove garlic, crushed
> 4 boneless, skinless single chicken breasts (about 1 ½ lb), cut into 2-inch pieces
> 1 green pepper, seeded and cut in chunks
> 1 cup sliced mushrooms
> 1 cup SALT-FREE tomato sauce or Fresh Tomato Sauce (see recipe, page 189)
> non-iodized salt and pepper to taste
> dried basil and dried oregano to taste
> LID-Safe Homemade Pasta (see recipe, page 103)

1. Combine onion, garlic, and chicken pieces in a single layer in an ungreased 2-quart oval or rectangular microsafe casserole. Cover with parchment paper.
2. Microwave covered on HIGH for 5 to 6 minutes, stirring twice. Chicken should just be losing its pink color. Drain off liquid. Add green pepper and mushrooms. Microwave covered on HIGH 2 to 3 minutes longer, until tender-crisp.
3. Add SALT-FREE tomato sauce and seasonings; mix well. Microwave covered on HIGH for 2 minutes, until sauce is hot. Let stand for 3 minutes.
4. Meanwhile, cook fettuccine conventionally. (I like to use fresh pasta, which only takes 1 to 2 minutes to cook.) Drain and rinse well. Top with chicken and vegetables.

Yield: 4 servings. Reheats well. Veggies will become soggy if frozen.

■ VEGETARIAN MAIN DISHES

Black Bean and Corn Casserole
(See recipe, page 109.)

Easy BBQ Chickpea Casserole
(See recipe, page 112.)

Easy Ratatouille
This versatile vegetarian dish makes a terrific sauce for LID-safe pasta or rice and is also excellent as a pizza topping. Use it as a filling for crêpes or egg white omelets. It's delicious when served chilled over salad greens and also makes a great dip or spread with LID-safe bread.

  2 medium eggplants (about 2 ½ lb in total), unpeeled
  2 medium onions
  1 green and 1 red pepper

1 medium zucchini
2 cups mushrooms
4 cloves garlic, minced
2 tbsp olive oil
non-iodized salt and pepper, to taste
½ tsp dried basil
¼ tsp dried oregano
3 tbsp balsamic or red wine vinegar
2 tbsp white sugar (or to taste)
2 – 5 ½ oz cans SALT-FREE tomato paste
½ cup water (approximately)

1. Spray a large heavy-bottomed pot with non-stick spray. Chop vegetables. Add oil to pot and heat on medium heat. Add vegetables and sauté for 10 to 12 minutes. If necessary, add a little water to prevent sticking.
2. Add seasonings, vinegar, sugar, tomato paste, and water. Simmer covered for 25 to 30 minutes, stirring occasionally. If mixture gets too thick, add a little water. Adjust seasonings to taste. Delicious hot or cold.

Yield: 8 to 10 servings. Keeps 1 week to 10 days in the refrigerator. Freezes well.

Easy Vegetarian Chili
(See recipe, page 112.)

Hearty Vegetable Stew
This satisfying stew is a winner! Vary the vegetables according to what you have on hand. Beans add fiber and protein. Enjoy without guilt!

1 tbsp olive oil
2 onions, chopped
1 red or green pepper
2 stalks celery

1 medium eggplant (do not peel)
2 medium zucchini (do not peel)
3 or 4 cloves garlic, minced
2 potatoes, peeled
3 ripe tomatoes
3 or 4 carrots, peeled and trimmed
28 oz can SALT-FREE tomatoes or 3 ½ cups Quick and Easy Tomato
Sauce (see page 192)
2 cups SALT-FREE canned or cooked kidney beans
non-iodized salt and ground pepper, to taste
2 tsp dried basil (or 2 tbsp fresh)

1. Heat oil on medium heat in a large, heavy-bottomed pot. Add onions and sauté for 5 minutes. Meanwhile, cut remaining vegetables into 1-inch chunks. Add red pepper and celery to onions. Reduce heat to low, cover and cook for 3 or 4 minutes. Add eggplant, zucchini, and garlic. Cook covered for another 5 minutes.

2. Add remaining ingredients and mix well. If using dried basil, add it now. If using fresh basil, add it at the end of cooking. Simmer partially covered for 25 to 30 minutes longer, until vegetables are done, stirring occasionally. Adjust seasonings to taste. If too thick, add a little water. If too thin, cook uncovered a few minutes longer.

Yield: 12 servings. Reheats and/or freezes well. Serve with LID-safe noodles, rice, or Basic Polenta (see recipe, page 46).

Variations:
- *Instead of zucchini, substitute 2 cups of butternut squash (peeled and cut into chunks).*
- *Replace potatoes with 8 to 10 new baby potatoes or 1 large sweet potato, peeled and cut into chunks.*

EGGPLANT 101

- Eggplant is available all year round and comes in a variety of shapes and sizes. The most common type is pear-shaped, with a dark purple skin. Most varieties are interchangeable in long-cooking dishes.
- Buy eggplant that's firm and heavy, with a smooth, glossy skin. Avoid those rough, spongy spots, and brown signs of decay.
- Small, slender eggplants have smaller seeds are sweeter and more tender, but larger ones are more practical.
- Eggplant is perishable and becomes bitter with age. It keeps about a week in a plastic bag in the refrigerator.
- Older eggplants have a tougher skin. Peel them when the recipe calls for long cooking. If the skin is tender, don't bother peeling it.
- Salting eggplant draws out bitter juices and excess moisture. Smaller varieties usually don't need to be salted before cooking. They also cook more quickly.

Homemade Pizza Sauce

(See recipe, page 108.)

Quick Matzo Pizza

(See recipe, page 108.)

CHAPTER SEVEN

DESSERTS

WHAT'S INSIDE

199

INGREDIENT SUBSTITUTIONS FOR BAKING

Substitutions and low-fat alternatives for LID baking.

For	Use
1 tbsp butter	1 tbsp canola or walnut oil or 1 tbsp LID-safe margarine
½ cup butter or margarine	½ cup LID-safe margarine or 3 tbsp canola oil plus ⅓ cup unsweetened applesauce, Prune Purée or a LID-safe fruit purée
1 cup butter or margarine	1 cup LID-safe margarine or ⅓ cup canola oil plus ⅔ cup unsweetened applesauce, Prune Purée or a LID-safe fruit purée
1 cup milk	1 cup orange juice, apple juice, black coffee, water, Rice Milk (page 56), Almond Milk (page 50), Coconut Milk (page 53) or SALT-FREE canned coconut milk

When you're off the LID, consider the following substitutions year-round for low-fat baking!

For	Use
1 egg	2 egg whites or 3 to 4 tbsp pasteurized egg whites (In baking recipes, too many egg whites may make baked goods dry. See "Advice from an Eggs-Pert" on page 204.) or ¼ cup mashed banana (Baked goods may be denser/heavier.) or combine 1 tbsp ground flaxseed with 3 tbsp water in a small bowl. Let stand until thick, 2 to 3 minutes. (Store flaxseed in the freezer to prevent rancidity.)
2 eggs (in baking)	3 egg whites or 6 tbsp pasteurized egg whites (Too many egg whites may make baked goods dry.)
salt	non-iodized salt or Kosher salt, finely ground
brown sugar	white sugar (Flavor may not be as intense. If desired, add a few drops of vanilla extract or maple flavoring.)
1 cup white sugar	½ cup white sugar plus ½ cup Splenda granular (Baked products may be denser, slightly drier than those made with only sugar.)
1 ounce (1 square) unsweetened chocolate	3 tbsp unsweetened pure cocoa powder plus ½ tbsp canola oil

SUBSTITUTING SHORTENING FOR BUTTER IN LID BAKING

Commercial vegetable-based shortening is made from an amalgam of vegetable oils, including soybean oil. Although soy protein is not allowed on the LID, soybean oil, in small amounts, is fine and the small amount of soybean oil that's in shortening is considered LID-safe (see Dr. Ain's Introduction). The following shortening substitution chart is for substituting Crisco shortening, as water must be added to Crisco. If you're using lard or other shortening, please consult the labels or manufacturer, as you'll be omitting the water.

For	Use
¼ cup butter or margarine	¼ cup Crisco shortening + ½ tsp water
⅓ cup butter or margarine	⅓ cup Crisco shortening + 2 tsp water
½ cup butter or margarine	½ cup Crisco shortening + 3 tsp water
⅔ cup butter or margarine	⅔ cup Crisco shortening + 4 tsp water
¾ cup butter or margarine	¾ cup Crisco shortening + 1 ½ tbsp water
1 cup butter or margarine	1 cup Crisco shortening + 2 tbsp water

Prune Purée

This is a fabulous fat substitute to use in baking. It's quick and easy to make, plus it's much cheaper than the commercial version. Prune Purée is packed with potassium and fiber. Prunes are also referred to as "dried plums."

2 cups pitted prunes (about 36)
1 cup hot water

1. Combine prunes and hot water in a bowl. Cover and let stand for 5 minutes, until plump. In a processor or blender, process prunes with water until smooth, about 1 minute. Scrape down sides of bowl several times.

Yield: About 2 cups. Store tightly covered in the fridge for up to 3 months, or freeze for 6 months.

Note: *This makes an excellent spread for matzo or LID-safe bread that's been toasted.*

EGG WHITE WISDOM

- Start with egg whites at room temperature when whipping egg whites. Make sure no yolk gets into the whites or they won't whip properly. Separate each egg white into a small bowl before adding it to the other whites. That way, if a drop of yolk gets into the white, it can be removed easily with a piece of egg shell.
- Use a glass, stainless, or copper bowl. Egg whites won't whip properly in a plastic bowl. Beaters must be clean and grease-free. Even a trace of grease will keep whites from whipping properly.
- If using a copper bowl, clean it with a little lemon juice and Kosher salt just before you use it.
- Cream of tartar helps egg whites reach maximum volume. Use ¼ tsp cream of tartar for every 4 egg whites. Omit cream of tartar when whipping egg whites in a copper bowl.
- If you don't have cream of tartar, substitute 1 tsp lemon juice for ¼ tsp cream of tartar.
- Beat egg whites with cream of tartar (or lemon juice) until foamy. Gradually beat in sugar, about 2 tbsp at a time. Properly beaten whites will be stiff but not dry. They should look glossy and you should be able to turn the bowl upside down without the whites falling out.
- No-guilt egg whites: Buy liquid egg whites in a carton. They're found in the refrigerator section at the supermarket. They're so convenient, and you don't have to feel bad about throwing out the yolks!
- Liquid egg whites are pasteurized, so you can use them in recipes that aren't cooked (e.g., homemade mayonnaise).

ADVICE FROM AN EGGS-PERT

- One large egg white measures 2 tbsp liquid. One large egg yolk measures 1 tbsp liquid.
- For 1 large egg, substitute 2 egg whites (or 3 to 4 tbsp liquid egg whites).
- For 2 large eggs, substitute 3 egg whites (or 6 tbsp liquid egg whites).
- Too many egg whites in a batter can have a drying effect, especially in low-fat baked goods. A good solution is to add 1 tsp canola oil for each egg yolk you're replacing. The extra fat helps tenderize baked goods by inhibiting the development of gluten in wheat flour that's created by mixing or beating batters.
- Leftover egg whites? They can be stored covered in the refrigerator for up to a month, or can be frozen successfully.
- Leftover egg yolks? You can refrigerate them for 2 or 3 days, or freeze them until you're no longer on your LID diet. Add a pinch of white sugar to yolks before freezing to prevent stickiness when thawed. You can also cook egg yolks and feed them to your dog or cat. It will make their coat shine.
- Frozen egg whites and yolks should be thawed overnight in the refrigerator. Never refreeze thawed frozen eggs.

■ CAKES

18-Carrot Cake (or Muffins)

Bake this "grate" cake in an oblong pan for everyday fare. For entertaining, use a fluted Bundt pan and drizzle with Lemon Glaze (see next page)—it's a gem!

18 mini carrots or 6 medium carrots (3 cups grated)
4 egg whites
½ cup canola oil
1 ¾ cups white sugar
2 tsp vanilla
½ cup unsweetened applesauce
2 ½ cups all-purpose flour
1 ½ tsp baking powder
1 ½ tsp baking soda
1 tbsp cinnamon
¼ tsp non-iodized salt
½ cup raisins
½ cup chopped, unsalted walnuts, if desired
Lemon Glaze (see page 206)

1. Preheat oven to 350ºF. Spray a 9-inch by 13-inch baking pan or a 10-inch Bundt pan with non-stick spray. Grate carrots, measure 3 cups, and set aside.
2. Combine egg whites, oil, sugar, vanilla, and applesauce in a mixing bowl or food processor. Beat until light, about 2 to 3 minutes. Add grated carrots and mix well.
3. Combine flour, baking powder, baking soda, cinnamon, and salt. Add to batter and mix just until flour disappears. Sprinkle raisins and nuts over batter and mix in with quick on/off pulses.

4.   Pour batter into prepared pan. Bake at 350ºF for 45 to 55 minutes, or until a toothpick inserted into the center of the cake comes out with no batter clinging to it. Cool for 15 to 20 minutes before removing cake from pan. Drizzle Lemon Glaze over cooled cake.

Yield: 12 to 15 servings. Freezes well.

Lemon Glaze:
1 ½ cups icing sugar
3 tbsp lemon juice
1 tsp lemon zest
½ tsp vanilla extract

1.   Combine all ingredients in a mixing bowl or food processor and blend until smooth. Drizzle over your favorite cake. If desired, sprinkle with unsalted chopped nuts.

Yield: Enough for a 10-inch Bundt cake.

Carrot Cupcakes: *Place batter in sprayed muffin pans. Bake at 375ºF for 20 to 25 minutes.*

Angel Food Cake
Fat-free, cholesterol-free, guilt-free! Read "Egg White Wisdom" (page 203). Use a tube pan with a removeable bottom for best results, not a Bundt pan.

¾ cup all-purpose flour
½ cup icing sugar
¼ tsp non-iodized salt
¾ cup white sugar
1 ½ cups egg whites (about 12), at room temperature
1 tsp cream of tartar
1 tsp vanilla

1. Preheat oven to 325ºF. Sift flour, icing sugar, and salt into a bowl. In the processor, process white sugar until fine, about 20 seconds.
2. In a large mixing bowl, beat egg whites with cream of tartar until soft peaks form. Gradually add finely ground sugar, beating at high speed until whites are stiff but not dry. Blend in vanilla. Using a rubber spatula, gently fold in flour mixture about ¼ cup at a time, just until blended.
3. Pour batter into an ungreased 10-inch tube pan and smooth the top. Use a knife to gently cut through batter to remove any large air bubbles. Bake on the middle rack at 325ºF for about 45 minutes, until golden. Immediately invert cake pan onto its raised feet (or hang it upside down over the neck of a bottle covered with aluminum foil; this will prevent the bottle from cracking or breaking). Let cake hang until completely cool.
4. To remove cake from pan, slide a thin-bladed knife or flexible spatula between pan and sides of cake. Push up the bottom of the pan; remove sides. Loosen around the center tube and the bottom of the pan. Carefully invert cake onto a large round serving platter. Cut with a serrated knife.

Yield: 12 servings. Cake can be frozen for 2 or 3 weeks if well wrapped.

Banana Cake

Use ripe bananas that are almost black for maximum flavor. Batter can also be baked as cupcakes (see next page).

> 3 large, very ripe bananas
> ¼ cup LID-safe margarine (e.g., Fleischmann's)
> or canola oil
> 1 cup white sugar
> 4 egg whites
> 1 tsp vanilla
> 1 tsp baking soda
> 1 tsp baking powder

2 cups all-purpose flour
½ cup orange juice
2 ounces dark, non-dairy chocolate, grated (about ½ cup), optional

1. Preheat oven to 350ºF. Spray a 7-inch by 11-inch Pyrex baking dish with non-stick spray.
2. Purée bananas in a food processor until smooth, about 20 seconds. Measure 1 ½ cups purée. Beat margarine or oil, sugar, egg whites, and vanilla until light, about 3 or 4 minutes. Blend in bananas. Add baking soda, baking powder, and flour. Drizzle orange juice over flour mixture. Process with several quick on/off turns, just until blended. Stir in grated chocolate, if using.
3. Spread batter evenly in prepared pan. Bake at 350ºF for 45 to 50 minutes, until golden and cake tests done.

Yield: 12 servings. Freezes well. If desired, top with Chocolate Glaze or Chocolate Frosting (see recipes, pages 212 and 213).

Banana Cupcakes: *Spoon batter into muffin pans lined with cupcake liners, filling them ¾ full. Bake in a preheated 375ºF oven for 20 to 25 minutes.*

Chocolate Angel Orange Cake

Follow directions for Angel Food Cake. At the end of Step 2, fold 2 tsp freshly grated orange rind and 2 ounces dark, non-dairy chocolate into batter.

Crazy Chocolate Cake

There are no eggs in this fast and fudgy chocolate cake, but no one will know unless you tell them!

1 ½ cups flour
1 cup white sugar
⅓ cup unsweetened pure cocoa powder (LID-safe)
1 tsp baking soda
½ tsp non-iodized salt
5 tbsp canola oil
1 tbsp white vinegar
1 tsp vanilla
1 cup cold water or coffee

1. Insert Steel Blade in food processor. Process flour, sugar, cocoa, baking soda, and salt for 10 seconds to blend. Add remaining ingredients and process 6 to 8 seconds longer, just until blended.
2. Pour into a sprayed 7- by 11-inch (or 9-inch square) baking pan. Bake in a preheated 350°F oven for 30 minutes.

Yield: 9 servings. Freezes well. Delicious with Peanut Butter Icing (see recipe, page 213), Chocolate Glaze (page 212), or Chocolate Frosting (page 213).

Variations:
- **Lazy Version:** *To save on cleanup, use the baking pan as your mixing bowl. Measure dry ingredients into baking pan; blend with a fork. Make depressions for the oil, vanilla and vinegar. Pour cold water or coffee over; mix well. Bake for 30 minutes at 350°F.*
- **Crazy Chocolate Cupcakes:** *Pour batter into muffin tins, which have been lined with paper liners. Bake at 375°F about 20 minutes, until done. Cool completely. Frost with Chocolate Glaze or Chocolate Frosting (see recipes on page 212 and 213).*

Lemon Loaf

Follow directions for Lemon Poppy Seed Cake (see below). Omit poppy seeds. In Step 4, divide batter in half and pour into two sprayed loaf pans. Bake in a preheated 350ºF oven for 40 to 45 minutes, until a cake tester inserted comes out clean. Immediately poke holes into the top of each loaf, using a wooden or metal skewer. Slowly drizzle hot syrup over the top of each loaf, letting them soak up the liquid. When cooled, remove carefully from pans and wrap well.

Lemon Poppy Seed Cake

Moist and lemony, with a slight crunch from the poppy seeds, this sin-free cake is a winner! You need two large, juicy lemons for this recipe: one for the cake and the other for the syrup. I used ¾ cup of liquid egg whites from the carton to make the cake, but you can substitute fresh egg whites if you prefer.

> 1 tbsp grated lemon zest
> ½ cup fresh lemon juice, divided
> ¾ cup orange juice
> ⅓ cup poppy seeds
> 6 egg whites
> ⅓ cup LID-safe margarine (e.g., Fleischmann's) or canola oil
> ⅔ cup unsweetened applesauce
> 1 ¼ cups white sugar
> 2 ½ cups all-purpose flour
> 2 tsp baking powder
> 1 tsp baking soda
> 6 additional tbsp white sugar

1. Grate rind from one large lemon and measure 1 tbsp zest. Squeeze juice from 2 lemons. You should have ½ cup juice. Reserve ¼ cup lemon juice for glaze. Combine remaining ¼ cup lemon juice with orange juice. Add poppy seeds and let soak for 15 minutes.

2. Preheat oven to 375ºF. Spray a 10-inch Bundt pan with non-stick spray.

3. In the processor or the large bowl of an electric mixer, combine egg whites, margarine or oil, applesauce, and 1 ¼ cups white sugar. Beat until light, about 3 minutes. Combine flour with baking powder and baking soda. Add to batter along with lemon zest. Pour poppy seed mixture over flour mixture. Mixture will bubble and fizz, but that's okay. Process with quick on/offs, just until flour disappears.

4. Pour batter into prepared pan. Bake at 350ºF for 50 to 60 minutes. A cake tester inserted near the center should come out clean.

5. Just before cake is done, prepare lemon syrup. Combine remaining 6 tbsp sugar with the reserved ¼ cup lemon juice and heat gently, stirring to dissolve sugar.

6. Remove cake from oven. Poke holes into the top of hot cake with a wooden or metal skewer. Use a brush and slowly brush half of the lemon syrup over the hot cake. It will take about 5 minutes. Let cake cool in pan for 15 to 20 minutes. Then, invert cake onto a large piece of foil and remove pan. Poke holes into the rest of the cake and slowly brush with remaining syrup. When completely cool, wrap cake in foil and let stand at least 12 hours before serving so that cake will absorb the lemon syrup.

Yield: 18 servings. Cake can be frozen.

Oat Bran Muffins
(See recipe, page 74.)

Yummy Apple Cake
This luscious cake will be even more moist the next day. For a large family, double the recipe and bake it in a 9- by 13-inch pan.

Batter:
4 egg whites
1 cup white sugar

1 tsp vanilla

½ cup canola oil

3 tbsp water or apple juice

1 ½ cups flour

2 tsp baking powder

½ tsp cinnamon

Filling:

6 large apples, cored, peeled and thinly sliced

⅓ to ½ cup additional white sugar (to taste)

2 tsp additional cinnamon

1. Preheat oven to 350ºF. Spray a 7-inch by 11-inch Pyrex pan with non-stick spray.
2. Batter: Beat egg whites, sugar, and vanilla until light. Beat in oil and blend well. Add water or apple juice, flour, baking powder, and ½ tsp cinnamon. Mix just until flour disappears.
3. Filling: In another bowl, mix apples with remaining sugar and cinnamon.
4. Assembly: Spread half of batter in pan. Spread apples evenly over batter. Top with remaining batter and spread evenly. (If you wet your spatula, the batter will be easier to spread.)
5. Bake at 350ºF for 50 to 60 minutes, until nicely browned.

Yield: 12 servings. If frozen, cake will become more moist. Just reheat it for 10 minutes at 350ºF.

■ FROSTINGS AND GLAZES

Chocolate Glaze

2 ounces dark, dairy-free chocolate

1 ½ cups confectioner's sugar

3 tbsp water or cold coffee
½ tsp vanilla

1. Place chocolate in a small microsafe bowl. (Make sure the bowl is completely dry.) Microwave uncovered on MEDIUM (50%) for 1 minute. Stir well. Microwave 30 to 60 seconds longer, until melted. Stir well; let cool.
2. Combine with remaining ingredients and blend until smooth. Drizzle over your favorite (non-dairy) chocolate cake.

Yield: Enough for a 9-inch square cake. Freezes well.

Chocolate Frosting: *Add ¼ cup LID-safe margarine (e.g., Fleischmann's). Process all ingredients in a food processor on the Steel Blade for 10 seconds, until smooth and blended (or place in a mixing bowl and beat well). Use to frost your favorite chocolate or banana cake.*

Peanut Butter Icing

1 ½ cups confectioner's sugar
6 tbsp Easy Low Iodine Peanut Butter (see recipe, page 250)
4 to 5 tbsp hot water (approximately)

1. Combine all ingredients in a food processor fitted with the Steel Blade. Process until smooth and blended, about 10 seconds, scraping down sides of bowl as needed.

Yield: Enough for a 7- by 11-inch oblong or 9-inch square cake. Freezes well.

■ PIES AND CRUSTS

A Basic Pie Crust

⅔ cup frozen shortening (e.g., Crisco)
2 cups flour
½ tsp non-iodized salt
1 tsp white vinegar
scant ½ cup ice water (about 3 ½ oz)

1. Steel Blade: Place chunks of shortening around the bottom of the processor bowl. Add flour and salt. Process with about 5 or 6 quick on/off turns, stopping to check texture, until mixture begins to look like coarse oatmeal. Do not overprocess. Add vinegar.
2. With machine running, add liquid in a steady stream through the feed tube just until the dough begins to gather around the blades, about 10 to 12 seconds after the liquid is added. Immediately remove dough from machine, press into a ball, divide in two and wrap each piece in foil or plastic wrap. (Each piece of dough should look like a large, thick hamburger patty.) Refrigerate dough for at least 1 hour before rolling out. (May be made 2 or 3 days in advance.)
3. Roll out dough on a lightly floured board (or preferably use a pastry cloth and a rolling pin stockinette cover). Roll equally in all directions, making sure to keep dough circular and mending cracks as they form. Roll about 2 inches larger than pie plate, about ⅛ of an inch thick.

Yield: Two 9-inch pie crusts. Freezes well.

Apple Crumb Pie

Follow directions for Basically Great Apple Pie (see below), but don't make a top crust and use only ½ cup white sugar to sweeten the apples. Prepare the following topping:

> ¾ cup flour
> ⅓ cup LID-safe margarine (e.g., Fleischmann's) or canola oil
> ½ cup white sugar
> ½ tsp cinnamon
> ¼ cup unsalted walnuts or pecans, optional

1. Steel Blade: Process all ingredients for topping about 8 to 10 seconds, until crumbly. Sprinkle topping over apples. Bake at 400ºF for 45 to 50 minutes, until filling is tender and topping is golden brown. Delicious! May be frozen. Serve warm or cold.

Note: *Any fruit may be substituted for the apple filling (e.g., peaches, pears, blueberries).*

Basically Great Apple Pie

> A Basic Pie Crust (see page 214) or double recipe of Soda Pastry (see page 221)
> 2 tbsp matzo meal
> 8 large apples, cored and peeled
> ½ to 1 cup white sugar (to taste)
> 1 tsp cinnamon
> 4 tbsp flour

1. Prepare pastry as directed. Roll out 1 portion of chilled pastry into a large circle and place in an ungreased 9-inch pie plate. Trim off overhanging edges. Sprinkle with matzo meal.

2. Insert Slicer in food processor. Cut apples to fit feed tube. Slice, using medium pressure. You should have 6 to 7 cups. The processor bowl should be nearly full. Combine apples in a mixing bowl with sugar, cinnamon, and flour.

3. Fill shell, mounding apples higher in the center. Roll out remaining dough, cut several slits. Place over apple filling. Trim away edges, leaving a half-inch border all around. Tuck under bottom crust. Flute edges.

4. Bake at 425ºF about 45 to 50 minutes. May be frozen baked or unbaked.

To freeze unbaked pie: *Do not cut slits in top crust. Wrap well and freeze. To bake, preheat oven to 450ºF. Bake for 15 minutes. Cut slits in top. Reduce heat to 375ºF and bake 45 minutes longer.*

Basically Great Peach Pie

Prepare as for Basically Great Apple Pie (see 215), but substitute 8 large peaches for apples. Peel by pouring boiling water over peaches, then place in cold water. Peel, cut in half, and remove pits. Slice. Increase flour to ⅓ cup, as peaches contain more moisture than apples.

Blueberry Apple Pie

Follow recipe for Basically Great Apple Pie (see page 215), but substitute the following filling:

3 to 4 apples, cored and peeled
1 ½ cups fresh or frozen blueberries (drained)
¾ to 1 cup white sugar
⅓ cup flour
1 tsp cinnamon

1. Insert Slicer in food processor. Cut apples to fit feed tube. Slice, using medium pressure. Combine with remaining filling ingredients and mix well. Assemble and bake as directed. May be frozen.

Cookie Crumb Crust

1 ¼ cups homemade LID-safe cookie crumbs (see Cookie Tips, page 233)
3 tbsp canola oil
2 tbsp orange juice
2 tbsp white sugar
½ tsp cinnamon

1. Preheat oven to 350ºF. Spray a 10-inch springform pan or 9-inch pie plate with non-stick spray. In a mixing bowl or food processor, combine crumbs, oil, orange juice, sugar, and cinnamon; mix well. Press mixture evenly into the bottom of prepared pan. Bake at 350ºF for 7 to 8 minutes. Cool completely.

Yield: 8 servings. Can be frozen.

Low Iodine Pie Crust

1 cup matzo meal
¼ cup white sugar
1 tsp cinnamon
¼ cup canola oil
2 tbsp orange juice

1. Combine all ingredients in a food processor fitted with the Steel Blade and mix until blended, about 20 seconds. Press into the bottom of a lightly sprayed 10-inch springform pan (or into the bottom and up the sides of a 9-inch pie plate. Bake at 375ºF for 15 minutes, until golden.

Yield: 1 pie crust (8 to 10 servings). May be frozen.

Meringue Tarts with Strawberries and Chocolate

These are heavenly. Perfect for entertaining!

Meringue:

4 large egg whites, at room temperature

½ tsp cream of tartar

dash of non-iodized salt

1 tsp vanilla extract

1 cup white sugar

Filling and Garnish:

4 cups fresh strawberries, hulled and sliced

3 to 4 tbsp additional white sugar

½ cup Easy Chocolate Syrup (see page 55) or 3 tbsp coarsely grated dark, dairy-free chocolate

1. Preheat oven to 250ºF. Cover a baking sheet with parchment paper or lightly greased aluminum foil.
2. Place egg whites in the large bowl of an electric mixer. Add cream of tartar, salt, and vanilla. Beat on medium speed until frothy, about 1 minute. With the mixer at high speed, gradually beat in sugar, 1 tbsp at a time. Continue beating until stiff, glossy peaks form, about 5 to 7 minutes. Mixture will look like marshmallow.
3. Drop meringue mixture from a rubber spatula onto prepared baking sheet, forming eight rounds about 3 to 4 inches in diameter (or spread to form one 10-inch circle). Build up sides with the back of a spoon to form a shell.
4. Bake at 250ºF for 1 hour. Turn the oven off and leave in oven for 1 to 2 hours to dry. Do not open oven door.

5. If meringues aren't going to be served immediately, remove them from the oven, let cool, then carefully peel off parchment paper. Store in a tightly covered dry container until needed.

6. Filling: Combine strawberries and sugar in a bowl and mix gently. (Can be prepared a few hours in advance and refrigerated.)

7. At serving time, fill meringues with sliced strawberries. Drizzle with Easy Chocolate Syrup (see recipe, page 55) or sprinkle with grated non-dairy chocolate.

Yield: 8 servings. Do not freeze.

Variation: *Drizzle Strawberry or Raspberry Purée (see recipe, page 232) over berries.*

Pine-Apply Pie

A Basic Pie Crust (see page 214) or double recipe of Soda Pastry (see page 221)
6 large apples, peeled, cored, and halved
14 oz can crushed pineapple, well drained
¾ cup white sugar (or to taste)
1 tsp cinnamon
¼ cup flour
2 tbsp matzo meal

1. Prepare pastry as directed. Chill dough while preparing filling.
2. Insert Slicer in food processor. Slice apples, using medium pressure. Transfer to a mixing bowl and combine with drained pineapple, sugar, cinnamon, and flour.
3. Roll out half of pastry on a floured pastry cloth, using a stocking cover for your rolling pin, or use a lightly floured board. Place in an ungreased 9-inch pie plate. Trim edges of pastry even with edges of pan. Sprinkle matzo meal in pie shell. Add filling, mounding it slightly higher in the

219

center. Roll out remaining pastry and cut several slits in it. Carefully place over filling. Trim dough, leaving a half-inch overhang. Tuck top crust under bottom crust. Flute edges. Brush crust with a little water and sprinkle with about 1 tsp sugar.

4. Bake at 425ºF for 10 minutes; reduce heat to 350ºF and bake 30 minutes longer, until golden.

Yield: 6 to 8 servings. Freezes well.

Rhubarb Pie

Yes, you CAN have rhubarb! See Dr. Ain's Introduction.

A Basic Pie Crust (see page 214) or double recipe of Soda Pastry (see page 221)
4 cups sliced rhubarb
1 ¼ cups white sugar (or to taste)
⅓ cup flour

1. Prepare pastry as directed. Chill before rolling.
2. Mix rhubarb with sugar and flour. (Rhubarb can be sliced in the food processor, using the Slicer.)
3. Roll out half of pastry on pastry cloth into a large circle about 2 inches larger than the pie plate. Transfer to an ungreased 9-inch pie plate. Trim off any overhanging edges. Fill with rhubarb filling. Roll out remaining pastry, cut slits in it and place over filling. Tuck top crust under bottom crust; flute edges. (Sprinkle with a little sugar, if desired.)
4. Bake at 425ºF for 40 to 50 minutes, until golden brown.

Yield: 8 servings. May be frozen.

Soda Pastry

1 cup + 1 tbsp flour
½ cup frozen LID-safe margarine
(e.g., Fleischmann's) or shortening
¼ cup ginger ale, 7-Up, or soda water
½ tbsp vinegar

1. Steel Blade: Process flour and margarine or shortening with on/off turns (about 2 to 3 seconds at a time) for 4 or 5 times, until the mixture begins to look like coarse oatmeal. Combine ginger ale with vinegar and add through feed tube while machine is running. Process just until the dough begins to gather in a mass around the blades, about 8 to 10 seconds. Do not overprocess.
2. Remove dough from machine and divide into 2 balls. (If dough is sticky, coat with a little extra flour.) Wrap in waxed paper or plastic wrap and chill in the refrigerator at least 1 hour, or overnight. The colder the dough, the easier it is to roll. Dough may be frozen baked or unbaked.

Yield: One 9-inch pie crust.

Note: *Recipe may be doubled in one batch successfully.*

■ CRISPS/COBBLERS

Blueberry Apple Crisp
This quick and easy recipe is perfect for inexperienced bakers. I teach it in my classes and everyone loves it.

Topping:
½ cup white sugar
¾ cup flour
½ cup canola oil

½ cup quick-cooking oats or LID-safe granola (see recipe for Great
Granola on page 47)
1 tsp cinnamon

Filling:
3 large apples, peeled and cored
2 cups fresh or frozen blueberries
¼ cup flour
⅓ cup white sugar
½ tsp cinnamon

1. Insert Steel Blade in food processor. Combine all ingredients for topping
   and process until crumbly, about 10 to 12 seconds. Empty contents of
   bowl onto a piece of waxed paper.
2. Filling: Slice apples. Combine with remaining filling ingredients and mix
   lightly. Spread evenly in a deep, ungreased 9-inch glass pie plate or 10-
   inch ceramic quiche dish, depressing the center slightly. Spread topping
   over filling and pat gently. Dish will be very full but mixture will reduce
   during cooking.
3. Microwave uncovered on HIGH for 12 to 14 minutes. Top will look
   cracked when done and fruit will be tender when pierced with a knife.
   Let stand for a few minutes before serving for topping to become more
   crisp. (Can be placed under the broiler briefly, if desired, but I never
   bother.) Serve warm or cold.

Yield: 8 to 10 servings.

- *It isn't necessary to defrost the berries before cooking.*
- *Topping can be prepared and kept in a plastic bag in the freezer. No need to
  thaw before using. A single serving can be made in a 10 oz glass custard cup
  and will take about 3 minutes on HIGH to microwave.*
- *One serving will take about 30 seconds uncovered on HIGH to reheat.*

Easy Apple Crisp

Filling:
6 medium apples, peeled, cored, and sliced
3 tbsp flour
¼ cup white sugar
1 tsp cinnamon

Topping:
1 cup flour
⅓ cup LID-safe margarine (e.g., Fleischmann's) or canola oil
½ cup white sugar
2 tsp cinnamon

1. Combine all ingredients for filling and mix well. Spread evenly in a deep, ungreased 9-inch glass pie plate or 10-inch ceramic quiche dish, depressing center slightly.
2. Steel Blade: Process all ingredients for topping 8 to 10 seconds, until crumbly. Do not overprocess. Sprinkle over apple mixture; pat down evenly. Microwave uncovered on HIGH for 10 to 12 minutes. When done, apples should be tender when pierced with a knife and top will be somewhat cracked. Serve warm or cold.

Yield: 8 servings. Can be frozen. (One serving will take 30 seconds uncovered on HIGH to reheat.)

Easy Pear Crisp
Prepare Easy Apple Crisp (see above), but substitute 4 cups sliced pears for apples; add 1 tsp lemon juice. Microwave time will be 12 to 14 minutes on HIGH.

Easy Rhubarb Strawberry Crisp

Combine 2 cups sliced rhubarb with 2 cups sliced strawberries, 1 cup white sugar and ¼ cup flour for the filling. Microwave time will be 12 to 14 minutes on HIGH. (Again, rhubarb is okay! See Dr. Ain's Introduction.)

Fruit Crisp

Follow recipe for Jumbleberry Crisp (see below), but substitute 6 to 7 cups of assorted sliced fresh (or frozen) fruits and/or berries (peaches, pears, nectarines, blackberries, etc.).

Jumbleberry Crisp

My cousin Nancy Gordon of Toronto gave me the idea for this fast and fabulous crisp based on her yummy Bumbleberry pie. I combined various berries, eliminated the crust, and this delectable dessert is the result. If you're missing one kind of berry, just use more of another. If using frozen berries, don't bother defrosting them. If you don't have apples, add extra berries!

Filling:

1 ½ cups strawberries, hulled and sliced
2 cups blueberries (fresh or frozen)
1 ½ cups cranberries and/or raspberries
2 large apples, peeled, cored, and sliced
⅓ cup flour (whole wheat or all-purpose)
⅓ cup white sugar
1 tsp cinnamon

Topping:

⅓ cup white sugar
½ cup flour (whole wheat or all-purpose)
¾ cup quick-cooking oats
1 tsp cinnamon
¼ cup canola oil

1. Combine filling ingredients; mix well. Spray a 10-inch glass pie plate or ceramic quiche dish lightly with non-stick spray. Spread filling ingredients evenly in dish.
2. Combine topping ingredients (can be done quickly in the processor). Carefully spread topping over filling and press down slightly.
3. Either bake at 375°F for 35 to 45 minutes until golden, or microwave uncovered on HIGH for 12 to 14 minutes, turning dish at half time. Serve hot or at room temperature.

Yield: 10 servings. Freezes well.

Time-Saving Secrets:
*   *Topping can be prepared ahead and frozen. No need to thaw before using.*
*   *Prepare crisp as directed, but use 6 to 7 cups assorted frozen berries and omit apples. Assemble in an aluminum pie plate, wrap well, and freeze it unbaked. When you need a quick dessert, unwrap the frozen crisp and bake it without defrosting at 375°F for about 45 minutes.*
*   *If you're making this dessert in the microwave, place a large microsafe plate or a sheet of parchment or waxed paper under the cooking dish to catch any spills.*

Peachy Crumb Crisp

Filling:
6 cups peeled, sliced peaches (or a combination of peaches, nectarines and plums)
1 tbsp lemon juice
¼ cup white sugar
¼ cup flour (whole wheat or all-purpose)
1 tsp cinnamon

Topping:
¼ cup white sugar
½ cup flour (whole wheat or all-purpose)
¾ cup quick-cooking oats
1 tsp cinnamon
2 tbsp canola oil
2 tbsp orange juice

1. Combine filling ingredients and place in a sprayed 10-inch ceramic quiche dish.
2. Combine topping ingredients and mix until crumbly. Sprinkle over fruit.
3. Bake at 400ºF for 45 minutes. If necessary, cover loosely with foil to prevent overbrowning.

Yield: 10 servings. Freezes well.

- **Blueberry Peach Crisp:** *Use 4 cups sliced peaches and 2 cups blueberries in the filling. Add 1 tsp grated orange zest if desired.*
- **Blueberry Nectarine Crisp:** *Use 4 cups sliced nectarines and 2 cups blueberries in the filling.*
- **Apple Crisp:** *Instead of peaches, use 6 cups sliced apples (e.g., McIntosh, Cortland, Spartan, Spy). Add ½ tsp grated nutmeg.*

Pecan Apple Crisp

Prepare Easy Apple Crisp (see recipe, page 223) as directed, but replace ½ cup flour with ½ cup finely chopped unsalted pecans in topping mixture.

■ FRUIT DISHES

Basic Baked Apples

4 medium baking apples, cored (e.g., McIntosh, Cortland, Spartan)
4 tbsp white sugar
1 tsp cinnamon

1. Either pierce skin of apples in several places with a fork or slice a band of skin ½ inch from the top of each apple in order for the steam to escape. Blend sugar and cinnamon. Fill center of each apple with cinnamon-sugar. Arrange in a circle in a 9-inch glass pie plate.
2. Cover with parchment paper and microwave on HIGH for 5 or 6 minutes, until apples are tender. (Calculate 5 to 6 minutes per pound; 3 apples make 1 pound.) Let stand covered for 3 to 4 minutes.

Yield: 3 to 4 servings.

- *One medium apple will be cooked in approximately 2 to 3 minutes. Two apples will take 3 to 4 minutes, depending on size and type of apple. Fill each apple with 1 tsp to 1 tbsp white sugar (to taste) and a pinch of cinnamon. Sugar substitute can also be used. Bake in a 10 oz glass custard cup or microsafe dessert dish.*
- *Apples can be filled with any mixture of your choice. Some suggestions are: cinnamon and unsalted chopped nuts, maple syrup, or raisins and unsalted chopped nuts.*

Dried Fruit Compote

1 ½ lb dried mixed fruit (prunes, apricots, etc.)
1 cup raisins
1 orange, sliced
½ lemon, sliced

¼ cup white sugar
½ tsp cinnamon
3 cups water or orange juice

1. Combine all ingredients in an 8-cup microsafe bowl. Place parchment paper under running water to make it flexible. You can then mold it around the bowl.
2. Microwave covered on HIGH for 15 minutes, stirring at half time.
3. Let stand covered until cool. Fruit will plump as it stands. Refrigerate. Serve chilled. Keeps about a week to 10 days in the refrigerator.

Yield: 6 to 8 servings.

Homemade Applesauce

Applesauce makes a wonderful accompaniment to potato latkes or a simple, delicious dessert on its own. My grandmother always added a ripe pear. Her applesauce was the best!

8 medium apples
1 Bartlett pear, optional
¼ cup water or apple juice
3 to 4 tbsp white sugar
1 tsp cinnamon

1. Peel and core the apples and pear. Cut them into chunks. Combine all ingredients in a large saucepan. Bring to a boil, reduce heat to simmer and cook partially covered for 20 to 25 minutes, until tender. (Or, microwave covered on HIGH for 6 to 8 minutes, until tender. Stir once or twice during cooking.)
2. Break up the applesauce with a spoon, or serve it chunky.

Yield: 6 servings. Freezes well.

Tips and Variations:

- *If you have a food mill, cook apples without peeling; wash well before cooking and discard stems. After cooking, put the mixture through a food mill. Applesauce will be a rosy pink.*
- *If using apple juice, use a minimum amount of sugar.*
- *If you want apples to keep their shape, add sugar after cooking, not before.*
- **Applesauce with Mixed Fruits Compote:** *Use your favorite combination of fruits (e.g., apples, pears, blueberries, strawberries, rhubarb, peaches, plums, nectarines) for a delicious dessert.*
- **Rella's Blueberry Applesauce:** *Add 2 cups of blueberries 5 minutes before end of cooking time.*
- **Pat Richman's Easiest Pink Applesauce:** *Add 16 oz of sliced strawberries or raspberries to 28 oz of applesauce. Serve in sherbet glasses. Pretty luscious! (Thanks to Devah Wine for sharing a "taste memory".)*

Pineapple Sherbet

Simply refreshing! This quick and delicious dairy-free sherbet is guaranteed to become a family favorite. Kids of all ages love it!

14 oz can pineapple (crushed or tidbits), with juice
2 tbsp pasteurized liquid egg whites, if desired

1. Open can of fruit and spoon the contents into ice cube trays. Freeze until nearly frozen, about 2 to 3 hours (or even overnight).
2. Just before serving, process fruit "ice cubes" in the food processor until the texture of sherbet. Scrape down the sides of the work bowl 2 or 3 times. Add egg white to mixture and process a few seconds longer. (The texture is smoother if you add the egg white.) Serve immediately.

Variations:
- *Any canned fruit in its natural juice (LID-safe) can be substituted for pineapple. Try canned peaches or apricots, for example.*
- *Other frozen ripe fruits or berries can be processed along with the pineapple (e.g., ripe bananas, strawberries, blueberries, mangoes).*

Poached Pears

The pears will be rosy pink. If your casserole doesn't have a cover, use parchment paper.

> 1 cup cranberry juice cocktail
> ½ tsp cinnamon
> 2 tbsp honey, optional
> 4 firm, ripe pears

1. Combine cranberry juice, cinnamon, and honey in a 1-quart microsafe casserole. Microwave uncovered on HIGH for 3 to 4 minutes, until boiling.
2. Meanwhile, peel pears; remove core from the bottom end. Don't remove stems. Place in hot juice, with the stem end pointing inwards.
3. Cover and microwave on HIGH for 5 to 6 minutes, turning pears over and rearranging them at half time. When done, pears will keep their shape but will be tender when pierced with a knife. Let cool, turning them over once or twice. Serve warm or chilled.

Yield: 4 servings. Do not freeze.

Stewed Prunes

> 1 ½ lb pitted prunes
> 1 cup Sultana raisins
> 3 cups water

¼ cup white sugar
½ lemon, thinly sliced
½ orange, thinly sliced

1. Combine all ingredients in an 8-cup microsafe bowl. Cover with parchment paper that has been placed under running water for a few seconds so you can mold it easily around the bowl.
2. Microwave covered on HIGH for 15 minutes, stirring at half time. Let stand covered until cool. Refrigerate. Serve chilled.

Yield: 6 to 8 servings. Keeps a week to 10 days in the refrigerator, or freezes well.

Stewed Rhubarb

Yes, you CAN have rhubarb. See Dr. Ain's Introduction.

4 cups peeled, sliced rhubarb
¼ cup orange juice or water
¾ cup white sugar, or to taste
1 cup sliced strawberries, if desired

1. Combine all ingredients except strawberries in a 3-quart microsafe casserole.* Cover and microwave on HIGH for 8 to 10 minutes, until tender, stirring at half time. Stir in strawberries. Let stand covered until cool. Refrigerate.

Yield: 6 servings.

Make sure to use a large enough bowl, as rhubarb mixture can boil over during cooking. Use parchment paper or a dinner plate if your casserole doesn't have a cover.

Strawberry or Raspberry Purée
Perfect over egg white omelets, pancakes, crêpes, fresh fruit, or cake.

> 2 cups ripe strawberries or raspberries, hulled
> 2 to 3 tbsp honey or white sugar
> 1 tsp orange juice, optional

1. Purée berries until smooth. A food processor does an excellent job. Sweeten with honey or sugar. Blend in orange juice. (Raspberries should be strained through a sieve to remove seeds.)

Yield: About 1 ½ cups. Can be frozen.

Summertime Fresh Fruit Compote
My daughter Jodi loves this recipe, even if I include rhubarb, which is not one of her favorites.

> 4 cups assorted fresh fruit (peaches, rhubarb, nectarines, plums, cherries, blueberries)
> 2 cups water
> ½ cup white sugar (to taste)
> 1 tbsp lemon juice

1. Peel peaches. Remove strings from rhubarb with a potato peeler. Don't bother peeling nectarines and plums. Remove pits from fruit. Cut larger fruit into chunks. Place in a 3-quart microsafe bowl. Cover with parchment paper that has been placed under running water for a few seconds so you can mold it easily around the bowl.
2. Microwave on HIGH for 10 minutes; stir. Microwave 4 or 5 minutes longer, until tender. Let cool; refrigerate.

Yield: 6 to 8 servings. Keeps about a week to 10 days in the refrigerator, or freezes well.

■ COOKIES AND MINI-CAKES

COOKIE TIPS:

* Bake cookies on the middle rack of your oven. When baking 2 pans of cookies at the same time, place racks so they divide the oven into thirds.
* For even baking, switch pans (top to bottom and front to back) for the last few minutes of baking.
* Not enough cookie sheets? While the first batch of cookies is in the oven, place the next batch on parchment or foil. When the first batch is baked, slide the parchment or foil (and cookies) off the pan. Cool the pan slightly, and then replace with the next batch of cookies.
* Process leftover or broken cookies on the food processor until fine. Use to make cookie crumbs for pie crusts, squares, and desserts. If you don't have a food processor, place cookies in a heavy plastic bag and crush with a rolling pin.
* Add ½ cup of leftover coconut pulp from Coconut Milk (see page 53) to your favorite cookie batter.

Almond Coconut Macaroons

Who would mind being marooned on a desert island if they could have these yummy macaroons to nibble on?

> 1 ½ cups blanched unsalted almonds
> 3 egg whites
> 1 tbsp lemon juice
> 1 cup white sugar
> 1 ½ cups grated coconut (see Note on following page)

1. Preheat oven to 350°F. Line cookie sheets with parchment paper.
2. Using the Steel Blade, process the almonds until finely ground, about 25 to 30 seconds. Transfer almonds to a small bowl and set aside. Wash the processor bowl and blade thoroughly. Dry them well.
3. Process the egg whites together with the lemon juice on the Steel Blade

for 1 minute, until light and foamy. Gradually add sugar through the feed tube while the machine is running. Process 1 minute longer.

4. Add coconut and ground almonds. Process 10 seconds longer to combine.

5. Drop mixture from a teaspoon onto parchment-lined cookie sheets. Bake at 350°F for 12 to 15 minutes, until set. These will be oatmeal-colored. Cool completely.

Yield: About 4 dozen. These freeze well, if you can hide them quickly enough!

Chocolate Macaroons: *Add 2 tbsp unsweetened pure cocoa powder to egg white mixture along with ground almonds and coconut.*

Note: *Some brands of packaged coconut contain salt. To grate fresh coconut, see recipe for Coconut Milk (page 53), Steps 1 to 3 inclusive.*

Chocolate Chewies

These are a chocoholic's delight. They're definitely addictive!

½ cup unsweetened pure cocoa powder (LID-safe)
2 cups confectioner's sugar
2 tbsp all-purpose flour
3 egg whites
½ tsp vanilla
2 cups finely chopped unsalted pecans or almonds

1. Preheat oven to 350°F. Line 2 baking sheets with aluminum foil and spray with non-stick spray (or line pans with ungreased parchment paper).

2. In the large bowl of an electric mixer, combine cocoa, icing sugar, and flour. Blend in egg whites on low speed. Increase to high speed and beat 1 to 2 minutes longer. Stir in vanilla and nuts.

3. Drop mixture by rounded spoonfuls onto prepared baking sheets, leaving about 2 inches between cookies. Press tops slightly with the bottom of a glass to flatten. Bake on middle rack at 350ºF for about 15 minutes, until set and crispy. Store in an airtight container.

Yield: 3 to 4 dozen cookies. Freezes well.

Oatmeal Cookies

    1 cup all-purpose flour
    1 cup rolled oats (regular or quick-cooking)
    ½ cup white sugar
    ½ tsp baking powder
    ½ tsp baking soda
    ¼ tsp non-iodized salt
    1 tsp cinnamon
    2 egg whites
    ¼ cup canola oil
    ⅓ cup corn syrup
    1 tsp vanilla
    ¾ cup raisins or dried cranberries, rinsed and drained

1. Preheat oven to 375ºF. Line a large baking sheet with foil and spray with non-stick spray.
2. In a large mixing bowl, combine flour, oats, sugar, baking powder, soda, salt, and cinnamon. Add remaining ingredients and stir well, until mixed.
3. Drop from a teaspoon 2 inches apart onto prepared pan. Bake on middle rack of oven at 375ºF about 10 minutes, until set and golden. Remove pan from oven and let cool. Cookies will become crisp upon standing.

Yield: About 3 ½ dozen cookies. These freeze well.

Old-Fashioned Sugar Cookies

Kids love to help by cutting out various shapes with cookie cutters. Cookies may vary in thickness, which affects the baking time, so be sure to check for doneness to prevent burning.

> 3 egg whites
> ¾ cup white sugar
> ½ cup canola oil
> 1 tsp vanilla
> ¼ cup orange or apple juice (or water)
> 2 tsp baking powder
> 3 cups flour
> additional sugar for dipping

1. Preheat oven to 375ºF. Beat egg whites, sugar, oil, and vanilla in a large bowl until light, about 1 to 2 minutes. Blend in juice. Stir in baking powder and flour, mixing to make a soft dough. (Don't overmix or dough will be tough.) Divide dough into 4 pieces.
2. Roll out each piece on a lightly floured surface into a rectangle about ⅛ inch thick. Cut dough into different shapes with assorted cookie cutters. Dip one side of each cookie lightly in sugar. Place sugar-side up on cookie sheets that have been lined with parchment paper or sprayed aluminum foil.
3. Bake at 375ºF for 8 to 10 minutes, until golden. Cool slightly, then remove from pans.

Yield: About 4 dozen. These freeze well.

Variations:

- *Dip top of each cookie in lightly beaten egg white, then in chopped nuts or sesame seeds combined with 2 tbsp white sugar.*

- *Dip top of each cookie in cinnamon-sugar.*
- **Chocolate Cookies:** *Increase sugar to 1 cup. Reduce flour to 2 ½ cups and add ½ cup unsweetened pure cocoa powder (LID-safe).*

Shortbread Cookies

Fleischmann's makes dairy-free unsalted margarine that's LID-safe (see chapter 1), which is available in most major supermarkets. It makes an excellent substitute for butter in these yummy cookies. If you can't find this margarine, don't make the cookies!

1 cup LID-safe margarine (see chapter 1), well-chilled or frozen
½ cup icing (confectioner's) sugar
¾ tsp vanilla
1 ½ cups all-purpose flour
½ cup cornstarch

1. Preheat oven to 350°F. Cut chilled or frozen margarine into chunks. In a food processor fitted with the Steel Blade, process margarine, icing sugar and vanilla until well-blended, about 1 minute. Scrape down sides of bowl. Add flour and cornstarch. Process with several quick on/off turns, just until dough begins to gather in a ball around the blades. Don't overprocess.
2. Shape dough into 1-inch balls (a small cookie scoop works well). Place on ungreased parchment-lined cookie sheets. Flatten in a criss-cross pattern with the floured tines of a fork, or press gently with the bottom of a glass that has been dipped in flour.
3. Bake on the middle rack at 350°F for 12 to 15 minutes. Edges of cookies should be slightly browned. Cool slightly before removing from pan.

Yield: Approximately 4 dozen. Freezes well.

Variations:

- **Nuts About Shortbread:** *Roll each ball of dough in a mixture of ¾ cup finely chopped pecans, walnuts, or almonds mixed with ¼ cup white sugar. Flatten in a criss-cross pattern with the floured tines of a fork.*
- **Shortbread Crescents:** *Shape dough into crescents. Dip in cinnamon-sugar or finely chopped nuts before baking.*

■ DARK CHOCOLATE (DAIRY-FREE CHOCOLATE)

Almond Bark

1 ¼ lb dark, dairy-free chocolate
2 cups toasted unblanched, unsalted almonds (or any nuts you like)

1. Line a cookie sheet with aluminum foil or parchment paper. Place broken-up chocolate in a dry 8 cup Pyrex measure. Microwave un-covered on MEDIUM for 2 minutes; stir. Microwave 1 to 2 minutes longer, stirring every minute, until chocolate is melted. Stir in almonds. Spread in a thin layer on foil. Freeze for 15 minutes, until hard. Break into chunks. Store in refrigerator.

Yield: About 1 ½ lb.

Chocolate-Dipped Strawberries
Elegant and easy!

2 dozen large strawberries
8 ounces dark, dairy-free chocolate, coarsely chopped
finely chopped, unsalted walnuts, if desired

1. Wash strawberries; do not remove stems. Gently pat dry with paper towels. Let stand to air-dry for 20 minutes. (Berries must be completely dry before dipping them in chocolate, or the chocolate will thicken and clump.) Line a large tray with parchment paper or aluminum foil.
2. In a dry, microsafe bowl, microwave chocolate uncovered on MEDIUM (50%) for 2 to 3 minutes, until melted, stirring every minute to prevent it from burning. Let cool until lukewarm, stirring occasionally.
3. Dip pointed end of strawberry ¾ of the way into melted chocolate. Allow excess chocolate to drip back into bowl. If desired, dip strawberries in chopped nuts. Arrange in a single layer on prepared tray. Repeat with remaining berries. If chocolate thickens, return it to the microwave and microwave on MEDIUM (50%) 30 seconds at a time to melt it.
4. Refrigerate berries about 20 minutes, until set.

Yield: 2 dozen. Do not freeze. These can be prepared up to 4 hours before serving time.

CHAPTER EIGHT

SNACKS

OR APPETIZERS!

WHAT'S INSIDE

SNACKS YOU CAN BUY IN A PACKAGE

As discussed in chapter 1, there are a myriad of SALT-FREE snacks available to consumers, in light of a demand for salt-free foods for people with hypertension. You can buy the following crunchy snacks in salt-free versions, and then use my recipes for seasoned non-iodized salts to make them appealing!

The following savory packaged snacks are available in SALT-FREE versions:
- Corn chips or tortilla chips;
- Some brands of potato chips (see my recipe for homemade potato chips);
- Nuts;
- Most main brands of crackers offer SALT-FREE varieties;
- Rice crackers of many varieties; and
- Popcorn (just buy it plain and air-pop, stove-top pop, or use a microwave popcorn maker).

GETTING CREATIVE WITH NON-IODIZED SALTS

You may find that you want to season your non-iodized salt, or need to alter the texture of a coarser salt (e.g. non-iodized Kosher salt), if you're using it. Seasoning is also perfect for snacks, or adding to a bag of no-salt crunchables. If you need a finer texture, you can place the salt in an electric coffee grinder for a few quick pulses until you reach desired texture, or you can use a mortar and pestle.

Note: *If you're using coarser salt, you may want to increase the quantity by up to one-third when adapting your favorite recipes.*

Cajun Seasoning

This sweet and spicy blend makes a delicious seasoning that is perfect for chicken or meat.

- 1 tbsp paprika
- 1 tbsp granulated garlic
- 1 tbsp granulated onion
- 1 tbsp white sugar
- 2 tsp non-iodized salt
- 2 tsp coarsely ground black pepper
- 2 tsp dried oregano (basil can be substituted)
- 2 tsp dried thyme

1. Combine seasonings in a bowl and mix well. Store in a covered container away from light and moisture. This will keep for 4 to 6 months.

Seasoned Salt

Multiply the ingredients for this mixture and keep it on hand as an all-purpose seasoning blend.

- ¼ cup non-iodized salt
- 2 tbsp freshly ground black pepper
- 2 tbsp granulated garlic
- 1 tbsp dried herbs (e.g., basil, oregano, thyme, and/or rosemary), or to taste
- 1 tsp paprika

1. Combine seasonings in a bowl and mix well. Store in a covered container away from light and moisture. This will keep for 6 months to a year.

Yield: About ⅓ cup.

SWEET PACKAGED SNACKS

You can buy the following sweet snacks for the LID diet:

- DAIRY-FREE chocolate (see below);
- Apple sauce;
- Dried fruits, such as raisins;
- Unsalted peanut butter for dipping apples, carrots, crackers, and rice cakes in. (You can dump unsalted peanut butter in a bowl, and mix it with non-iodized salt and then spoon it back in the jar. Also see my homemade peanut butter recipe, on page 250.);
- Nuts you can honey roast at home with non-iodized salt; and
- Natural sorbets, with no food coloring or dairy.

A Note About Chocolate: *Sadly, you'll need to stay away from milk chocolate while on the low iodine diet. However, non-dairy chocolate, such as dark chocolate, is LID-safe. A designation of "pareve" means your chocolate is dairy-free. The pareve designation was originally designed for people who keep Kosher, and need to separate meat from dairy. That said, it's important to note that the designation of "Kosher" chocolate does not mean it's necessarily pareve, as there are many dairy products that can still be Kosher.*

■ HOMEMADE CARBS (CHIPS AND CHIP SUBSTITUTES)

Crisp Lasagna Chips

You'll flip over these chips! Plus, they're perfect party fare. Whenever you make lasagna, cook up some extra noodles for this super snack. Pass-ta chips, please!

8 oz lasagna noodles (½ of a 1 lb package)
3 tbsp olive or canola oil
2 tbsp water

¼ cup matzo meal
non-iodized salt, to taste
dash of paprika

1. Cook lasagna noodles according to package directions. Drain well. Carefully separate the noodles and place them on clean towels in a single layer. Pat lightly to absorb extra moisture.
2. Preheat oven to 400ºF. Spray 2 baking sheets with non-stick spray.
3. Combine oil and water in a small bowl. Brush both sides of noodles lightly with oil mixture. Cut into 1 inch strips. Arrange a single layer of noodles on baking sheets. (You'll have to make several batches.) Combine matzo meal with salt and paprika. Sprinkle lightly over noodles.
4. Bake uncovered at 400ºF for 15 to 20 minutes, until crisp and golden. Shake pan once or twice during baking and watch carefully to prevent burning. When cool, store in an airtight container for a week or two (if you can resist them!).

Yield: About 12 dozen (12 servings). If desired, reheat for 4 or 5 minutes at 350ºF before serving.

Homemade Potato Chips

Packaged chips that are salt-free can be hard to find. Also, they're full of fat, calories, and sodium. These crunchy munchies are easy and guilt-free! When you're off the LID, you may prefer these to regular chips.

1 to 4 medium Idaho potatoes
non-iodized salt to taste
dried basil, oregano, garlic powder, and/or cayenne, if desired

1. Scrub potatoes thoroughly; dry well. Slice paper thin, either in the processor or by hand. You should get about 24 slices from each potato.

2.   Microwave Method: Place 12 slices at a time on a microsafe rack. Sprinkle lightly with desired seasonings. Microwave on HIGH for 4 minutes, or until dry and crunchy. Watch carefully because cooking time depends on moisture content of potatoes. If necessary, microwave 30 seconds longer and check again. Repeat until crispy. Repeat with remaining potato slices.

3.   Conventional Method (for a large batch): Preheat oven to 450ºF. Spray a baking sheet lightly with non-stick spray. Place potato slices in a single layer on pan. Sprinkle lightly with seasonings. Bake at 450ºF about 15 to 20 minutes, until crispy and golden.

Yield: Calculate ½ potato (about 12 chips) as 1 serving. Do not freeze.

Tips:
- *These are best eaten within a few days. The fresher, the better (they never last very long at my house)!*
- *Next time you have a snack attack, just remember that 15 potato chips (1 oz) contain 10 grams of fat and 150 calories. Homemade potato chips are "cheaper by the dozen" in more ways than one!*

Lavasch (Flatbread)

These are a great alternative to packaged crackers. They're perfect with soups, salads, dips, and spreads.

    1 cup flour
    ½ cup rolled oats (regular or quick-cooking)
    ¼ tsp non-iodized salt
    1 tbsp onion flakes
    2 tbsp sesame seeds
    ¼ tsp garlic powder
    2 tbsp canola oil
    6 tbsp water

Optional Toppings: *Sesame seeds, non-iodized Kosher salt, dill weed, dried basil, and/or dehydrated onion flakes.*

1. Preheat oven to 475°F. Line 2 baking sheets with aluminum foil and spray with non-stick spray. Combine flour, rolled oats, seasonings, and oil in the processor. Process until mixed. Slowly add water through the feed tube and process until mixture gathers together into a crumbly mass. Remove dough from processor and press it together to form a ball. Divide into 18 smaller balls.

2. On a floured surface, roll out each piece of dough as thin as possible into long strips. During the rolling process, sprinkle dough with desired toppings, pressing the toppings into the dough with the rolling pin. (Alternately, use a pasta machine to roll out dough.)

3. Bake at 475°F for 5 to 6 minutes, until crisp and golden.

Yield: 18 pieces. Store in an airtight container.

Matzo-Style Flatbread

If matzo isn't readily available in your area, here's how to make your own. These crunchy, cracker-like flatbreads are absolutely addictive!

> 2 cups flour
> ½ tsp non-iodized salt (or to taste)
> ¾ cup cold water (approximately)

1. Preheat oven to 475°F. Place two large baking sheets in the oven to heat up. (Oven racks should be on the second and fourth positions from the bottom of the oven.) Dust work surface with flour.

2. Place flour and salt in the processor bowl fitted with the Steel Blade. Gradually add water through the feed tube while the machine is running. Process until dough forms a ball, about 20 to 30 seconds. If dough seems dry, drizzle in a little extra water.

3.   Remove dough from processor and divide into 8 balls. Flatten each ball between your hands. Roll out each piece of dough into a circle with a rolling pin. Re-roll a second time into a circle about 7 inches in diameter, rolling dough as thinly as possible.

4.   Armed with a fork in each hand, quickly prick dough all over to make at least 100 holes. Turn dough over and pierce to make another 100 holes. (Don't worry—no one's counting!)

5.   Carefully transfer matzos to baking sheets, using tongs. Bake for 2 to 3 minutes per side, until lightly browned and crisp. Cool on a rack.

Yield: 8 matzos. Store in airtight containers.

Variations:
- *After transferring the unbaked matzos to baking sheets, brush each one with a little olive oil and sprinkle with non-iodized salt. Bake as directed.*
- *If desired, sprinkle unbaked matzos with your favorite dried herbs (e.g., basil, oregano, thyme, rosemary). Sesame seeds also make a tasty topping.*

Whole Wheat Pitas

For hors d'oeuvres, make miniature pitas. Baking time will be 5 to 6 minutes.

1 tsp white sugar
¼ cup warm water (110°F)
1 package active dry yeast (about 1 tbsp)
1 ½ cups all-purpose flour
1 ½ cups whole wheat flour (approximately)
1 tsp non-iodized salt
2 tsp additional white sugar
1 cup lukewarm water
1 tsp canola oil

1.   Dissolve 1 tsp sugar in ¼ cup warm water. Sprinkle yeast over water

and let stand for 8 to 10 minutes, until foamy. Stir to dissolve.

2. Combine flours, salt, additional sugar, and yeast mixture in processor. Process on the Steel Blade for 8 to 10 seconds. Pour lukewarm water and oil through feed tube while machine is running. Process until dough is well-kneaded and gathers in a mass around the blades, about 1 minute. If machine begins to slow down, add 2 or 3 tbsp additional whole wheat flour.

3. Transfer dough to a lightly floured surface. Knead dough for 2 minutes by hand, until smooth. Divide dough into 16 balls. Roll each ball into a circle about ¼ inch thick. Cover with a towel and let rise for ½ hour. Roll out thinly once again and let rise ½ hour longer.

4. Preheat oven to 500ºF. Place pitas on a lightly greased or sprayed baking sheet. Bake about 6 to 8 minutes, or until puffed up and golden. Inside of pita will be hollow. Cool on a rack. To fill, make a slit along one edge of pita and stuff as desired.

Yield: 16 pitas. These freeze very well.

■ DIPS AND SPREADS

Avocado Guacamole

Although avocados are high in fat (½ cup mashed avocado contains 185 calories and 17.6 grams fat), the main fat is monounsaturated oleic acid, which is also concentrated in olive oil. Take heart! Avocados benefit arteries, dilate blood vessels, and lower LDL (or "bad") cholesterol. It's believed that they also block many carcinogens.

> 2 medium-size ripe avocados (preferably Hass avocados)
> 2 tbsp fresh lime or lemon juice
> 2 cloves garlic, crushed
> 1 medium-size ripe tomato, chopped
> 4 green onions, chopped

½ of a red pepper, chopped
dash of cayenne
non-iodized salt and ground pepper, to taste

1. Coarsely mash avocado. (A potato masher works well, or use quick on/
    offs in your processor.) Immediately sprinkle with lime or lemon juice.
    Combine with remaining ingredients and mix lightly. Transfer to a
    serving dish. Place plastic wrap directly on the guacamole to prevent
    discoloration. Serve chilled as a dip with SALT-FREE corn chips, matzo
    or any LID-safe food. A scoop of guacamole can also be served as a salad
    over assorted greens.

Yield: About 2 cups. Mixture keeps for a day or two in the refrigerator. Do not
freeze.

Easy Low Iodine Peanut Butter

2 cups unsalted peanuts*
2 to 3 tbsp canola oil, if desired
non-iodized salt, to taste

1. Steel Blade: Place peanuts in a processor bowl. Process for approximately
    2 ½ minutes, stopping machine several times to scrape down sides of
    bowl. If you want a smoother texture, add oil. Blend in salt to taste.

Yield: About 1 cup. Store in refrigerator.

Chunky Peanut Butter: *Add ½ cup peanuts to peanut butter. Process 6 to 8
seconds longer.*

*You may use any nuts you wish instead of peanuts, so long as they're salt-free. For
a real delicacy, try UNSALTED cashews.*

Eggplant Spread #1
Cooking eggplant in water prevents it from changing color and turning dark.

> 1 onion, halved
> 1 tbsp oil
> 1 eggplant (about 1 ½ lb), peeled
> water to cover
> 1 small clove garlic
> non-iodized salt and ground pepper, to taste
> juice of ½ lemon
> 1 tomato, cut in chunks

1. Steel Blade: Process onion with 2 or 3 quick on/off turns, until coarsely chopped. Sauté in oil until golden, about 5 minutes.
2. Slicer: Cut eggplant to fit feed tube. Slice, using medium pressure. Place in a saucepan and add just enough water to cover. Cook covered until tender, about 10 to 15 minutes. Drain well.
3. Steel Blade: Drop garlic through feed tube while machine is running. Process until minced. Scrape down sides of bowl. Add remaining ingredients and process with several quick on/off turns, just until blended. Serve as a spread with Lavasch (see recipe, page 246) or Matzo-Style Flatbread (see page 247).

Yield: About 1 ½ cups. May be frozen.

Eggplant Spread #2

> 2 eggplants (about 1 ¼ lb each)
> 1 medium onion or 6 green onions (scallions)
> 2 cloves garlic
> 1 green pepper, seeded and cut in chunks
> ½ stalk celery, cut in chunks

251

1 tomato, quartered
non-iodized salt and ground pepper, to taste
1 to 2 tbsp oil (or to taste)
1 tbsp vinegar or lemon juice
½ tsp white sugar

1.   Cut eggplants in half lengthwise and place cut-side down on a broiling rack. Preheat broiler. Broil eggplant about 4 inches from heat for 15 minutes. Do not turn. (This gives the eggplant a charred flavor.) Let cool.
2.   Steel Blade: Process onion with garlic until minced, about 6 to 8 seconds. Add green pepper and celery and process with 2 or 3 quick on/off turns, until coarsely chopped. Remove eggplant pulp from skin with a spoon and add with remaining ingredients to processor bowl. Process with 3 or 4 quick on/off turns, just until mixed. Adjust seasonings to taste. Refrigerate or freeze.

Yield: About 3 cups.

Garlic Spread

4 large, fresh, plump heads of garlic
½ cup SALT-FREE chicken broth or broth from Free Chicken Soup
(see recipe, page 83)

1.   Place one of the garlic heads on a cutting board and cover it with a dish-towel. (This keeps garlic from flying around like ammunition!) Bang the bottom of a heavy frypan or pot onto the cloth-covered garlic. Remove the cloth; separate the cloves and pick out any easily removed papery skins. Cover garlic again with the towel and hit it again a couple of times. Discard any remaining skins. Repeat with remaining heads of garlic.

2. Place peeled garlic and broth in a small saucepan and bring to a boil. Reduce heat, cover tightly and simmer gently until tender, about 20 minutes. If necessary, add 2 or 3 tbsp more broth if most of it has evaporated.

3. Spread garlic thickly on matzo or LID-safe bread product.

Yield: 4 or more servings. Do not freeze.

Hummus (Middle Eastern Chickpea Spread)

¼ cup loosely packed parsley
2 cloves garlic
19 oz can SALT-FREE chickpeas, drained and rinsed
⅔ cup olive oil
½ cup tahini (sesame seed butter or paste)
6 tbsp fresh lemon juice
1 tsp non-iodized salt
freshly ground pepper
½ tsp cumin (or to taste)
3 tbsp additional olive oil, to garnish
paprika, to garnish (optional)

1. Steel Blade: Make sure that parsley and processor bowl are dry. Process parsley until minced. Set aside. Drop garlic through feed tube while machine is running. Process until minced. Add chickpeas, ⅔ cup olive oil, tahini, lemon juice, salt, pepper and cumin. Process until smooth.

2. Spread mixture on a large flat serving plate. Drizzle with remaining oil and sprinkle with reserved parsley. May be garnished with paprika. Serve chilled or at room temperature with Whole Wheat Pitas (see recipe, page 248). Also good as a dip with raw or steamed vegetables, Lavasch (see page 246) or Matzo-Style Flatbread (see page 247).

Yield: About 2 cups. Hummus keeps about a week, refrigerated. Do not freeze.

Tips and Variations:
- *Although tahini is fairly high in fat, it contains important nutrients such as zinc, iron, and calcium, and also provides flavor. Tahini can be found in supermarkets, Middle Eastern groceries, or health food stores.*
- *To lower the fat in tahini, discard the oil that comes to the top of the jar. Less fat, same flavor!*
- **Skinnier Hummus:** *Replace half the oil with ⅓ cup drained chickpea liquid.*

Red Lentil Pâté

Savor the flavor of "almost liver" without guilt or cholesterol. Thank you, Suzi Lipes.

> 2 cups red lentils, picked over and rinsed
> 4 cups SALT-FREE vegetable broth or homemade Vegetable Broth (see recipe, page 134) or water
> 1 tbsp olive oil
> 2 large onions, chopped
> 3 or 4 cloves garlic, minced
> 1 tsp each dried basil, oregano, and thyme
> ½ cup fresh parsley, minced
> ¼ cup matzo meal (plus 2 tbsp to coat the pan)
> ½ tsp non-iodized salt (to taste)
> freshly ground pepper (to taste)
> 2 tsp fresh lemon juice or balsamic vinegar
> 1 tsp Oriental sesame oil

1. Cook lentils in broth or water until tender, about 25 minutes. Do not drain. Let cool, then mash.

2. Heat oil in a large non-stick skillet. Add onions, garlic, and dried herbs. Sauté on medium heat until brown, stirring often. Add to lentils along with remaining ingredients; mix well.

3. Preheat oven to 350°F. Spray a 9- by 4-inch loaf pan with non-stick spray. Sprinkle pan with 2 tbsp matzo meal, lightly coating bottom and sides of pan. Spread lentil mixture in pan. Bake uncovered for 30 minutes, until set. When cool, un-mold and refrigerate. Best served at room temperature.

Yield: 12 slices. Leftovers keep 3 to 4 days in the refrigerator. Freezing intensifies the flavor of the herbs.

Roasted Garlic

Roasted garlic is so soft that you can spread it on toasted bread like butter, so mild that you can eat it without risking killer garlic breath! Its mellow flavor enhances salad dressings, pastas, soups, sauces, dips, or even mashed potatoes. Why not roast several heads? They taste great hot or cold!

2 large, fresh, plump heads of garlic

1. Preheat oven to 375°F. Cut a ¼ inch slice from the top of each head of garlic. Discard any loose, papery skins. Wrap each head of garlic in foil.

2. Bake for 30 to 40 minutes, until very soft. (Garlic can be baked in a toaster oven for 25 to 30 minutes, or cooked on the BBQ.) Cool slightly.

3. Squeeze cloves out of the skin directly onto matzo, or LID-safe bread products.

Yield: 2 or more servings. Do not freeze. Leftovers can be store for 4 or 5 days in a tightly closed container in the fridge.

Smoky Eggplant Dip

The peppers or onions are baked, not fried, in this tasty dish. Thanks to Ethel Cherry for sharing her scrumptious recipe with me.

2 medium eggplants (about 2 lbs)
2 green peppers
1 large onion, peeled and sliced
1 clove garlic
1 to 2 tbsp olive oil
1 tbsp vinegar
½ tsp white sugar
1 tsp cumin, or to taste
¼ cup chopped coriander/cilantro or parsley
4 drops liquid smoke (available in health food or gourmet stores)
non-iodized salt and ground pepper, to taste

1. Preheat oven to 400°F. Place eggplants, peppers, and onions (no need to cut them first) on a sprayed baking sheet and bake until soft. Peppers and onions will take 30 minutes; eggplants will take 45 to 50 minutes.
2. Cut eggplants in half and scoop out flesh. Drain well; discard the skin. Cut peppers in half and discard seeds.
3. Combine all ingredients except eggplant in the processor; chop coarsely. Add eggplant; process with quick on/offs. Transfer to a serving bowl and refrigerate.

Yield: About 4 cups. Serve with toasted pita chips, flatbread, or SALT-FREE crackers. Mixture keeps 4 or 5 days in the fridge.

Super Salsa

This fresh salsa makes a delicious dip for SALT-FREE corn chips, matzo, or any other LID-safe food. It's also great with grilled chicken or burgers.

4 large, ripe tomatoes (or 8 Italian plum tomatoes), finely chopped
2 cloves garlic, crushed
½ cup coriander/cilantro or parsley, minced
1 jalapeno pepper, seeded and minced
2 tbsp fresh basil, minced (or 1 tsp dried)
¼ cup green onions, chopped
2 tsp olive oil, to taste
2 tbsp fresh lemon juice, to taste
non-iodized salt and ground pepper, to taste
dash of cayenne
1 tbsp SALT-FREE tomato paste, optional

1. Combine all ingredients except tomato paste and mix well. (The processor does a quick job of chopping the vegetables.) If mixture seems watery, add the tomato paste. Season to taste.

Yield: About 3 cups. Salsa keeps for 2 to 3 days in the refrigerator in a tightly closed container.

Tips and Variations:
- *Italian plum tomatoes make a thicker salsa than regular tomatoes because they're firmer, with less seeds and juice.*
- *Don't rub your eyes after handling hot peppers. It's a smart idea to wear rubber gloves. Don't forget to remove the gloves before touching your eyes or you'll be yelling "eye, eye, eye!"*
- **Black Bean Salsa:** *Add a pinch of cumin and 1 cup SALT-FREE canned or cooked black beans to Super Salsa.*

- **Salsa Salad Dressing:** *Combine leftover salsa with a little SALT-FREE tomato juice in the food processor. Process with 6 or 8 on/off turns.*
- **Salsa Chicken in a Snap:** *Cut several large squares of cooking parchment or aluminum foil. Place a boneless chicken breast on each square. Top each one with a spoonful of salsa. Seal packets tightly. Arrange on a baking sheet and place in a preheated 400ºF oven for 20 to 25 minutes. Easy and good!*

■ OTHER STUFF (WHEN YOU'RE FEELING PECKISH!)

Microwave Pumpkin Seeds

Use the seeds from a fresh pumpkin and roast your own! The pumpkin pulp can be cooked and used as a substitute for squash.

1 cup pumpkin seeds
1 tbsp olive oil
non-iodized salt, to taste

1. Wash pumpkin seeds very well; pat dry. Place a double layer of microsafe paper towels in a 7-inch by 11-inch oblong microsafe casserole. (Paper towels must NOT be made from recycled paper because they could ignite.) Sprinkle seeds evenly on top of paper. Microwave uncovered on HIGH for 5 to 6 minutes. Remove paper towels from casserole, letting seeds slide back into bottom of dish.
2. Microwave seeds on HIGH 4 to 6 minutes longer, stirring halfway through cooking. Seeds should be dry but still white in color. Let stand for 5 minutes to continue drying.
3. Add olive oil to seeds. Sprinkle with non-iodized salt and mix well. Store uncovered.

Roasted Red Peppers

Roasted yellow and orange peppers also taste great! Very delicious, very versatile.

1. Preheat the broiler or BBQ. Broil or grill peppers until their skin is blackened and blistered. Keep turning them until they're uniformly charred.
2. Immediately put them into a brown paper bag or covered bowl and let cool.
3. Scrape off the skin using a paring knife. Rinse quickly under cold water to remove any bits of charred skin. Pat dry. Cut in half and discard stem, core, and seeds. If desired, cut peppers into strips. These freeze beautifully.

Chef's Secrets:
- *If you have a gas stove, roast one pepper at a time over a high flame using a long-handled fork. Buy peppers in the fall when prices are cheap. Broil or barbecue a large bunch of them at one time, then cool and peel. Discard the stem, core, and seeds. Freeze in small containers.*
- *An easy way to freeze these is to place roasted pepper halves or pieces in a single layer on a foil-lined baking sheet. When frozen, transfer them to freezer bags and store in the freezer until needed. Defrost as many as you need at one time.*
- *Roasted pepper strips are absolutely wonderful in sandwiches. Puréed roasted red peppers add a smoky taste to salad dressings, soups, sauces, dips, and spreads.*

Tomato and Basil Bruschetta

An easy company appetizer from Nancy Gordon and Hart Peikoff. Serve on matzo or a LID-safe bread product.

3 large tomatoes, diced (2 cups)
½ cup fresh basil (or 1 tsp dried)
1 clove garlic, crushed

non-iodized salt and ground pepper, to taste
matzo or a LID-safe bread product
1 large clove garlic, halved
1 to 2 tbsp olive oil (preferably extra virgin)

1. Combine tomatoes, basil, garlic, non-iodized salt, and pepper in a bowl; cover and refrigerate.
2. If using LID-safe bread, cut it into 12 slices, about 1 inch thick. Broil until lightly browned on each side. (Matzo doesn't need to be broiled.)
3. Rub the cut side of a garlic clove on one side of bread or matzo. Dip pastry brush in water, then in olive oil. Lightly brush oil on bread or matzo. (Can be prepared in advance.)
4. Top with tomato mixture. Serve immediately.

Yield: 12 appetizers. Do not freeze.

■ SWEET STUFF

All of the desserts in the previous chapter will make great snacks. But these will be easy to take with you, and don't require a fork!

Almond Bark
(See recipe, page 238.)

Almond Coconut Macaroons
(See recipe, page 233.)

Best Blueberry Orange Muffins
(See recipe, page 66.)

Chocolate Chewies
(See recipe, page 234.)

Crazy Chocolate Cake/Cupcakes

(See recipe, page 209.) Make cake as described, but bake in muffin/cupcake tins, filling them ⅔ full.

Magical Carrot Muffins

(See recipe, page 72.)

Oatmeal Cookies

(See recipe, page 235.)

Old-Fashioned Sugar Cookies

Kids love to help by cutting out various shapes with cookie cutters. (See recipe, page 236.)

Shortbread Cookies

(See recipe, page 237.)

CHAPTER NINE

CHILDREN'S MENU

WHAT'S INSIDE

263

■ EASY BREAKFASTS

These are selected items from our Breakfast chapter that we think your kids will especially like!

Apple Cinnamon Pancakes
(See recipe, page 61.)

Basic Sweet Egg White Omelet
(See recipe, page 60.)

Best Blueberry Orange Muffins
(See recipe, page 66.)

Blueberry Pancakes
Follow recipe for Easy Pancakes (see page 64), but stir ½ cup fresh or frozen blueberries into batter.

Broccoli Pancakes
(See recipe, page 96.)

Carrots-for-Breakfast Pancakes
(See recipe, page 62.)

Crêpes
(See recipe, page 63.)

Easy Pancakes
These are very easy to mix up and make an excellent breakfast or brunch dish. (See recipe, page 64.)

Egg Whites, Any Style and Ketchup

(See recipe for Egg Whites, page 60.) Most children prefer egg whites and won't touch the yolks. Now you don't have to argue! Serve with Homemade Low Iodine Ketchup (page 183).

Homemade Applesauce

Applesauce makes life easy when you're trying to find something for a child to eat! (See recipe, page 228.)

Homemade Low Iodine Ketchup

(See recipe, page 183.) A lot of children will want this as a topping on everything.

Magical Carrot Muffins

(See recipe, page 72.)

No-Knead Cinnamon Coffee Cake (Babka)

(See recipe, page 72.)

Old Fashioned Oatmeal

(See recipe, page 48.)

Regular Cream of Wheat

(See recipe, page 47.)

Salty Cream Of Wheat

Some children prefer their Cream of Wheat with salt—similar to grits. Make Cream of Wheat as directed on page 47, but serve with non-iodized salt sprinkled on top. If they like it, they'll eat it!

Zucchini-for-Breakfast Pancakes
(See recipe, page 65.)

■ PIZZA

Even though it has no cheese, nothing succeeds like pizza!

Homemade Pizza Sauce
(See recipe, page 108.)

Pizza Potato Skins
(See recipe, page 99.)

Quick Matzo Pizza
Quantities are for one pizza. Just multiply the ingredients by the number of pizzas you need. (See recipe, page 108.)

■ PEANUT BUTTER

Many children eat nothing but peanut butter and turn out fine! If your child is one of them, then the LID is no big deal. Of course, peanut allergies are a problem these days, so you may need an alternative if your child has nut allergies, or is attending a school where peanut products are banned.

Easy Low Iodine Peanut Butter
(See recipe, page 250.)

■ HAMBURGER FARE

Best Meatballs
(See recipe, page 166.)

Old-Fashioned Hamburgers
(See recipe, page 115.)

Red Hot Chili
(See recipe, page 174.)

Savory Shepherd's Pie
(See recipe, page 117.)

■ NOODLES AND DUMPLINGS

Fast Pasta with Veggies
Use one pot to cook the pasta and the veggies! It doesn't get much easier or faster than this. (See recipe, page 101.)

LID Soup Dumplings
(See recipe, page 131.)

Noodle Apple Bake
(See recipe, page 105.)

Noodle Bake
(See recipe, page 104.)

Pasta with Pesto and Tomatoes
This is guaranteed to become a family favorite! For variety, use differently shaped LID-safe pasta. (See recipe, page 105.)

Quick and Easy Tomato Sauce (Vegetarian Spaghetti Sauce)

Excellent over LID-safe noodles. (See recipe, page 192.)

■ CHILD-FRIENDLY CHICKEN

Breaded Chicken Fillets

(See recipe, page 148.)

Chicken Fingers

(See recipe, page 151.)

Chicken Spaghetti Soup

(See recipe, page 80.)

Doug's Quick Chicken Dinner

(See recipe, page 153.)

Grilled Chicken Kabobs

(See recipe, page 154.)

Mini Grilled Chicken Kabobs

(See recipe, page 160.)

Quicky Chicky with Fettuccine

(See recipe, page 193.)

■ HOT STUFF THEY'LL EAT

Apricot Candied Carrots

(See recipe, page 138.)

Corn on the Cob
(See recipe, page 141.)

Country Vegetable Soup
(See recipe, page 125.)

Yum-Yum Potato Wedgies
(See recipe, page 101.)

■ EASY SNACKS AND TREATS

Almond Bark
(See recipe, page 238.)

Almond Coconut Macaroons
(See recipe, page 233.)

Banana Cupcakes
(See recipe, page 207 to 208.)

Chocolate Glaze
(See recipe, page 212.)

Chocolate Chewies
(See recipe, page 234.)

Crazy Chocolate Cupcakes
(See recipe, page 209.)

Crisp Lasagna Chips
(See recipe, page 244.)

Homemade Potato Chips
(See recipe, page 245.)

Oatmeal Cookies
(See recipe, page 235.)

Old-Fashioned Sugar Cookies
Kids love to help by cutting out various shapes with cookie cutters. (See recipe, page 236.)

Peanut Butter Icing
(See recipe, page 213.)

Shortbread Cookies
(See recipe, page 237.)

Tomato and Basil Bruschetta
(See recipe, page 259.)

CHAPTER TEN

NUTRITIONAL ANALYSIS CHART FOR LOW IODINE FOODS

Since so many of you will be adapting these recipes, relying on store-bought items, and/or mixing and matching ingredients, the following chart provides nutrition information for an extensive variety of foods you'll use while on your low iodine diet. This chart does not include any foods that contain iodine, and calculates:

- Fats (saturated and unsaturated fats);
- Sugars (total sugars if sugar is added, or natural sugars, as in fructrose, which is the natural sugar in fruit, and maltose, the natural sugar in grains);
- Fiber (*SOL means the food is high in soluble fiber); and
- Sodium (the sodium content is based on the sodium content of foods containing no salt, or based on the average use of adding non-iodized salt to home cooked foods, or items normally purchased in the store, such as baked goods).

When you see the term "na" it means the information on the particular nutrient for a particular food item was "not available." This is not the same as "zero." When you see the term "t" it means the nutrient is present only in trace amounts, such as is sometimes the case with fats.

For those of you who are hypothyroid while on this diet, aim for foods with a higher fiber content (4 grams or higher) as well as foods that are lower in saturated fats. For those of you with diabetes, use the "sugars" information in this chart to help you with your meal planning, and choose foods lower in saturated fats and higher in fiber. For those of you with high blood pressure, use the "sodium" information to help you choose lower sodium foods, as well as foods lower in saturated fats.

Remember, many of the foods on this chart will be lower in sodium since we provide salt-free versions of many store-bought items.

All the information in this chart is based on existing data from the United States government, and from brand-name food manufacturers. Also consulted were: the U.S. Department of Agriculture (USDA) National Nutrient Database; numerous journal articles that analyzed the nutrient content of various foods; and various computer- and Internet-based sources, including Diet Expert, Food Count and Nutribase.

Note: This nutritional analysis model was adapted from an existing Food Counter model, created by Lynn Sonberg for the book, *Foods that Combat Heart Disease* (2005).

Food	Serving Size	Calories	Fat/Sat. Fat (gm)	Poly/Mono Unsaturated Fat (gm)	Fiber (gm)	Sugars (gm)	Sodium (mg)
BEEF*							
Brisket, braised**	3 oz.	185	8.6/3	.3/3.4	0	0	44
Chuck roast, baked**	3 oz.	250	16/6	.6/7	0	0	58
Eye of the round**	3 oz.	165	7/2.6	.3/3.7	0	0	49
Flank steak**	3 oz.	176	8.6/3.7	.3/3	0	0	54
Hamburger (3 oz. = 1 patty)							
Beef patty, cooked from frozen	3 oz.	240	17/6.5	2.5/.27	0	0	55
Extra lean, broiled medium	3 oz.	218	14/5.5	na	0	0	61
Extra lean, broiled well done	3 oz.	225	13.4/5	na	0	0	64
Lean, broiled medium	3 oz.	231	16/6	na	0	0	69
Lean, broiled well done	3 oz.	238	15/6	.62/7.3	0	0	na
Regular, broiled medium	3 oz.	246	17.5/7	na	0	0	65
Regular, broiled well done	3 oz.	248	16.5/6.5	na	0	0	na
Steak							
Porterhouse, broiled	3 oz.	254	19/7	.7/8	0	0	54
Rib-eye, broiled	3 oz.	188	10/3.7	na	0	0	na
Round tip, roasted	3 oz.	186	9.6/3.6	.3/3	0	0	35
T-bone, broiled	3 oz.	238	16.5/6.4	.6/7	0	0	56
Sirloin, broiled	3 oz.	211	12/5	.4/6	0	0	62
Tenderloin, roasted	3 oz.	239	16/6	.8/8.7	0	0	48

* Based on normal use of non-iodized salt to taste.
** Trimmed to $^1/_8$" fat, all grades.

Food	Serving Size	Calories	Fat/Sat. Fat (gm)	Poly/Mono Unsaturated Fat (gm)	Fiber (gm)	Sugars (gm)	Sodium (mg)
BEEF* (continued)							
Variety meats							
Brain, pan-fried	3 oz.	167	13.5/3	2/3	0	0	134
Heart, simmered	3 oz.	149	5/1.4	.8/.8	0	0	50
Liver, pan-fried	3 oz.	185	7/2.3	.6/.6	0	0	77
Tongue, baked	3 oz.	237	17/7.5	.6/8.5	0	0	55
BEVERAGES							
Coffee							
Brewed, decaf	1 cup	4.7	0/0	0	0	0	5
Brewed, regular	1 cup	4.7	0/0	0	0	0	5
Instant, decaf	1 cup	3.5	0/0	0	0	0	2
Instant, regular	1 cup	3.6	0/0	0	0	0	1
Fruit Juices							
Apple juice, canned, no sugar, w/ added Vit. C	1 cup	117	.27/.04	.08/.01	.25	na	7
Apple juice, canned, no sugar, no added Vit. C	1 cup	117	.27/.05	.08/.01	.25	10.9	7
Apple juice, concentrate, no sugar, w/added Vit. C	1 cup	112	.24/.04	.07/t	.24	27.6	7
Apple juice, concentrate, no sugar, or added Vit. C	1 cup	112	.24/.04	.07/t	.24	27.6	7
Apricot nectar, w/added Vit. C	1 cup	140.5	.23/.01	na	1.5	36	na
Apricot nectar, no added Vit. C	1 cup	140.5	.23/.01	na	1.5	34.6	na

* Based on normal use of non-iodized salt to taste.

Food	Serving Size	Calories	Fat/Sat. Fat (gm)	Poly/Mono Unsaturated Fat (gm)	Fiber (gm)	Sugars (gm)	Sodium (mg)
BEVERAGES Juices (cont.)							
Grape juice, concentrate, w/added sugar, Vit. C	1 cup	127.5	.23/.07	.7/t	.25	26.12	17
Grape juice, unsweetened, w/added Vit. C	1 cup	152	.2/.1	na	.25	na	na
Grape juice, unsweetened, w/o added Vit. C	1 cup	154	.2/.06	.05/t	.25	37.6	8
Grapefruit juice, pink, fresh	1 cup	93	.25/.03	.05/.03	na	22.7	2
Grapefruit juice, white, fresh	1 cup	96	.25/.03	.05/.03	.25	22.5	2
Grapefruit juice, sweetened, canned	1 cup	115	.22/.03	.05/.03	.25	27.57	5
Grapefruit juice, unsweetened, canned	1 cup	94	.25/.03	.05/.03	.25	21.88	2
Grapefruit juice, concentrate, sweetened	1 cup	118	.25/t	na	.25	na	na
Grapefruit juice, concentrate, unsweetened	1 cup	101	.32/.05	.07/.04	.25	23.79	2
Lemon juice, bottled	1 tbsp.	13	.04/t	.01/t	.06	.36	3
Lemon juice, from 1 lemon	1 fruit	12	0/0	0/0	.19	1.13	0
Lime juice, bottled	1 tbsp.	3.2	.04/t	.01/t	.06	.21	2
Lime juice, from 1 lime	1 fruit	3.2	.04/t	.01/t	.06	.64	1
Mango nectar, canned	1 cup	146	.3/.1	t/t	1.8	31	0
Orange juice, fresh	1 cup	112	.5/.06	.09/.09	.05	20.8	2
Orange juice, canned, unsweetened	1 cup	105	.35/.04	.08/.06	.5	20.9	5
Orange juice, from carton, unsweetened	1 cup	109.5	0/0	0/0	.5	169	0

Food	Serving Size	Calories	Fat/Sat. Fat (gm)	Poly/Mono Unsaturated Fat (gm)	Fiber (gm)	Sugars (gm)	Sodium (mg)
BEVERAGES Juices (cont.)							
Orange juice, from concentrate, diluted	1 cup	112	.15/.01	.03/.02	.5	20.9	2
Orange-grapefruit, canned, unsweetened	1 cup	106	.25/.03	.03/.02	2.5	20.9	2
Passion fruit, carton	1 cup	152	0/0	0/0	na	36	42
Peach nectar, canned, w/added Vit. C	1 cup	134	.05/t	t/t	1.5	34.7	na
Peach nectar, canned, w/o added Vit. C	1 cup	134	.05/t	t/t	1.5	34.7	na
Pineapple, unsweetened, w/added Vit. C	1 cup	140	.2/.01	.07/.02	.5	33.95	3
Pineapple, unsweetened	1 cup	140	.2/.01	.07/.02	.5	33.95	3
Pineapple, from concentrate	1 cup	130	.07/t	.02/t	.5	31.4	3
Orange-grapefruit juice	1 cup	80	0/0	0/0	.4	19	0
Pineapple-orange juice, canned	1 cup	125	0/0	0/0	.25	29	8
Tropical blend, carton	1 cup	120	0/0	0/0	0	22	15
Prune juice, bottled or canned	1 cup	182	.07/t	.08/.05	2.6	42.1	10
Strawberry-banana-orange juice, carton	1 cup	126	0/0	0/0	2.6	27	14
Cranberry apple drink, bottled	1 cup	165	0/0	0/0	.24	44.1	17
Cranberry grape drink, bottled	1 cup	137	.25/.08	.05/.01	.24	34.3	7
Cranberry juice cocktail, bottled	1 cup	144	.25/.02	.11/.03	.25	34.2	5
Cranberry juice cocktail, low-calorie, bottled	1 cup	45	0/0	0/0	0	10.9	7
Grape juice drink, canned	1 cup	125	0/0	0/0	.25	31.9	3

276

Food	Serving Size	Calories	Fat/Sat. Fat (gm)	Poly/Mono Unsaturated Fat (gm)	Fiber (gm)	Sugars (gm)	Sodium (mg)
BEVERAGES Juices (cont.)							
Lemonade, concentrated, diluted	1 cup	99	0/0	0/0	0	25.9	7
Limeade, concentrated, diluted	1 cup	101	0/0	0/0	.25	22.1	5
Vegetable Juices							
Carrot juice, fresh or no salt	1 cup	94	.35/.06	.16/.01	1.8	9.23	na
Tomato juice, low sodium, no salt	1 cup	41	.15/.02	.1/.03	2	9.2	na
Vegetable juice w/tomato, no salt	1 cup	46	.2/.03	.1/.03	2	9.2	na
Teas							
Green tea, brewed	1 cup	2.4	0/0	0/0	0	na	na
Herbal tea, brewed	1 cup	2.3	0/0	t/t	0	.47	2
Iced tea, with lemon (Nestle)	1 cup	88	.7/.05	0/0	0	18	0
Tea (black), brewed	1 cup	2.4	0/0	0/0	0	0	7
Tea, instant, sweetened, w/added Vit. C	1 cup	88	t/t	.02/t	0	177.6	8
IODINE-FREE BREADS*							
Cinnamon raisin bagel	3" diameter	192	1.2/.2	.4/.29	1.3	36.6	348
Multigrain bagel	3" diameter	148	3.5/.5	2/.8	4	8	430
Oat bran bagel	3" diameter	145	.7/.1	.27/.1	2*SOL	.93	289
Plain, enriched bagel	3" diameter	157	1/.12	.39	1.3	.55	304
Whole wheat bagel	3" diameter	151	2.5/.5	1/.9	5.3	7	630
Homemade biscuit	2 ¼" dia.	212	16/4	4/7	.9	45	586
Bread crumbs, homemade	½ cup	395	5.7/1.2	2.2/1	2.4	6.7	791
Bread stuffing, homemade	½ cup	178	8.6/1.7	2.6	3	2.1	543
Cornbread stuffing, homemade	½ cup	179	9/1.8	3.8	3	21.9	455

*Baked with non-iodized salt by you or your bakery.

Food	Serving Size	Calories	Fat/Sat. Fat (gm)	Poly/Mono Unsaturated Fat (gm)	Fiber (gm)	Sugars (gm)	Sodium (mg)
IODINE-FREE BREADS* (cont.)							
Branola bread	1 slice	89	1.2/.3	na	1.4	na	na
Cinnamon bread	1 slice	69	.9/.1	na	.6	na	na
Cracked wheat bread	1 slice	65	1/.23	.2/.57	1.4	14.8	161
French or Viennese bread	1 med. slice	68.5	.75/.16	.4/.77	.75	.15	390
Fruit and nut bread	1 slice	217	10/2	na	1	na	na
Granola bread	1 slice	89	1.2/.3	na	1.4	na	na
High fiber, reduced-calorie bread	1 slice	60	.7/.2	na	3	na	na
High protein bread	1 slice	64	.6/.1	na	.8	.27	104
Italian bread	1 med. slice	54	.7/.17	.27/.16	.5	.17	117
Low-gluten bread	1 slice	73	1.4/.2	na	1.5	na	na
Mixed grain (7-grain, whole grain)	1 slice	65	1/.2	.25/1	1.7	na	na
Mixed grain, reduced-calorie bread	1 slice	52.5	.6/.1	na	3	na	122
Oat bran bread	1 slice	71	1.3/.2	.5/.47	1.3 *SOL	2.31	na
Oat bran bread, reduced-calorie	1 slice	46	.7/.1	.38/.15	2.7 *SOL	.81	81
Oatmeal bread	1 slice	72	1.2/.4	.46/.42	1	2.2	162
Oatmeal bread, reduced-calorie	1 slice	48	.8/.14	.3/.18	na	43.3	89
Pita, white, enriched	1 large, 6.5"	165	.72/.1	.3/.06	1.3	.78	322
Pita, whole wheat	1 large, 6.5"	170	1.7/.3	.67/.2	5	.5	340
Potato bread	1 slice	69	.9/.1	na	.6	na	na
Raisin bread	1 slice	71	1.1/.3	.17/.59	1	5.7	101
Rice bran bread	1 slice	66	1.2/.5	.47/.44	1.3	1.26	119

*Baked with non-iodized salt by you or your bakery.

Food	Serving Size	Calories	Fat/Sat. Fat (gm)	Poly/Mono Unsaturated Fat (gm)	Fiber (gm)	Sugars (gm)	Sodium (mg)
IODINE-FREE BREADS* (cont.)							
Rye bread, light	1 slice	52	1.6/.2	.2/4	1.2	.08	211
Rye bread, reduced calorie	1 slice	46	.6/.08	.17/.15	3	.53	93
Rye bread, snack-sized	1 slice	18	.23/.04	.05/.09	.4	.02	46
Sunflower seed bread	1 slice	75	1.4/.4	na	1.6	na	na
Wheat bread, including wheatberry	1 slice	65	1/.2	.22/.43	2.8	1.37	133
Wheat germ bread	1 slice	73	.8/.2	.18/.35	.6	1.04	155
White bread, reduced calorie	1 slice	48	.6/.12	.12/.24	2.2	1.09	104
Whole wheat bread	1 slice	69	1.2/.25	.28/.47	2	5.56	148
Muffin, bran	1 muffin	168	5/.8	na	4.4 *SOL	na	na
Muffin, corn	1 muffin	180	7/1.3	3.5/1.7	na	na	333
Muffin, plain	1 muffin	169	6.5/1.3	3.2/1.5	1.5	2	26
Taco unsalted, corn, large	6 ½" dia.	98	4.7/.7	na	1.6	na	na
Taco unsalted, corn, medium	5" dia.	62	3/.4	na	1	19	na
Taco unsalted, flour, large	10" dia.	286	15/3.6	na	2	34	na
Tacos unsalted, flour, regular	7" dia.	173.5	9/2.2	na	1	31	na
Tortilla unsalted, corn, large	8" dia.	73	.8/.1	na	1.7	na	na
Tortilla unsalted, corn, medium	6" dia.	42	.5/.1	na	1	na	na
Tortilla unsalted, flour, large	10" dia.	218	5/1.2	na	2	na	na
Tortilla unsalted, flour, medium	8" dia.	140	3/.8	na	1.4	na	na
Tortilla unsalted, whole wheat, lar.	8" dia.	109	.7/.1	na	3	na	na
Tortilla unsalted, whole wheat, med	7" dia.	103	3.1/.65	1.2/.7	3.3	29	na

*Baked with non-iodized salt by you or your bakery.

Food	Serving Size	Calories	Fat/Sat. Fat (gm)	Poly/Mono Unsaturated Fat (gm)	Fiber (gm)	Sugars (gm)	Sodium (mg)
COLD CEREALS (Iodine-free)*							
100% Bran (Post)	¹⁄₃ cup	83	.6/.08	0/0	8.3 *SOL	7	120
All Bran (Kellogg's)	½ cup	79	.9/.2	.03/.2	9.7 *SOL	4.7	73
Bran Flakes (Kellogg's)	¾ cup	95	.6/.1	.32/.14	4.6 *SOL	4.9	207
Frosted Shredded Wheat (Post)	1 cup	190	1/0	.5/0	6 *SOL	11	0
Granola, homemade	1 cup	570	30/6	.13/9.3	13 *SOL	24.5	na
Kretschmer Honey Crunch Wheat Germ	1 ²⁄₃ cup	52	1/.15	na	1.5	3.3	na
Generic Shredded Wheat	1 ¼ cup	170	1/0	.5/0	6	1	na
Puffed Rice	1 cup	56	.07/.01	0/0	.24	12.6	0
Puffed Wheat	1 cup	44	.14/.02	0/0	.5	9.55	0
Shredded Wheat (Post)	2 biscuits	156	.5/.09	na	5.3	na	na
Shredded Wheat, spoon-sized (Post)	1 cup	167	.5/.1	0/0	5.6	.44	na
Shredded Wheat and Bran (Post)	1 ¼ cup	197	.8/.1	0/0	8 *SOL	.59	na
HOT CEREALS (Iodine-free)**							
Corn grits, regular, white	1 cup	145	.5/.07	.19/.12	.5	31.5	540
Corn grits, regular, yellow	1 cup	145	.5/.07	.2/.1	.5	.24	540
Cream of rice	1 cup	127	.24/.05	.06/.07	.25	.05	2
Cream of wheat, instant, plain	1 cup	149	.5/.09	.32/.08	1.4	.17	10
Cream of wheat, regular	1 cup	126	.5/.08	.26/.06	1	.15	146
Oat bran	½ cup	146	3/.6	.2/.04	6 *SOL	.57	2
Oatmeal (regular)	½ cup	157	2/.36	.62/.75	2.8 *SOL	13	261

* There are several cold cereals that have no salt; these are representative of only a few.
** You add your own salt when cooking these cereals, which can be non-iodized. Sodium content based on added non-iodized salt.

Food	Serving Size	Calories	Fat/Sat. Fat (gm)	Poly/Mono Unsaturated Fat (gm)	Fiber (gm)	Sugars (gm)	Sodium (mg)
CHICKEN*							
Fried (batter-dipped) breast	1 breast	218	11/3	2.6/4.6	.25	na	231
Fried (batter-dipped) drumstick	1 drumstick	115	6.7/1.8	1.6/2.8	.13	3.6	116
Fried (batter-dipped) thigh	1 thigh	238	14/4	2.03/3.5	.26	4.7	150
Fried (batter-dipped) wing	1 wing	94	6/1.7	1.5/2.6	.09	3.2	93
Fried (flour-coated) breast	1 breast	131	5/1.5	1.2/2	.06	.97	45
Fried (flour-coated) drumstick	1 drumstick	71	4/1	.94/1.6	.03	.47	26
Fried (flour-coated) thigh	1 thigh	162	9/2.5	2.1/.6	.06	1.97	55
Fried (flour-coated) wing	1 wing	61	4/1.15	.94/1.7	.02	.45	15
Ground patty, cooked	4 oz. patty	143	8/2.3	na	0	na	na
Roasted breast (meat only)	1 breast	86	2/.5	.4/.64	0	0	38
Roasted breast (meat & skin)	1 breast	114	4.5/1.2	.96/1.7	0	0	41
Roasted dark meat	1 cup	269	12.6/3.4	3.2/5	0	0	130
Roasted leg	1 leg	109	5/1.3	1.1/1.7	0	0	52
Roasted light meat	1 cup	242	6/1.7	1.4/2.1	0	0	108
Roasted thigh	1 thigh	91	6/1.6	1.3/2.1	0	0	46
Roasted wing	1 wing	61	4/1.14	.87/1.6	0	0	17
Giblets, fried	1 cup	402	19.5/5.5	4.9/6.4	0	6.3	164
Giblets, simmered	1 cup	228	7/2	1.2/1.4	0	0	97
Liver, simmered	1 cup	220	7.6/2.6	1.5/1.7	0	0	95

* Assuming normal use of non-iodized salt, LID-safe coatings, and no butter or margarines.

Food	Serving Size	Calories	Fat/Sat. Fat (gm)	Poly/Mono Unsaturated Fat (gm)	Fiber (gm)	Sugars (gm)	Sodium (mg)
CRACKERS*							
Matzo	1 matzo	115	2/.4	na	.3	na	na
Matzo, dietetic	1 matzo	91	.4/0	na	.1	na	na
Matzo, whole wheat	1 matzo	100	.4/.07	na	3.4	na	na
Melba toast, bran	1 cracker	16	.4/.1	na	.2	na	na
Melba toast, plain	1 cracker	19.5	.16/.02	.06/.04	.3	.05	na
Melba toast rounds	4 rounds	47	.4/0	na	.8	na	na
Melba toast, wheat	1 cracker	19	.12/.08	.05/.03	.4	3.82	na
Melba toast, whole grain	1 cracker	16	.4/.1	na	.2	.2	na
Multigrain, wheat	13 crackers	120	5/0	na	3	na	na
Rice cracker	2 crackers	30	0/0	na	0	na	na
DIPS**							
Avocado	2 tbsp.	46	4.4/.7	na	1.4	na	na
Babaghanouj (eggplant dip)	2 tbsp.	47	4/.5	na	.8	na	na
Bean	2 tbsp.	40	1/.5	na	2.4 *SOL	na	na
Black bean	2 tbsp.	20	0/0	na	1 *SOL	na	na
Guacamole	2 tbsp.	46	3/.4	1/1.1	0	4	na
Hummus	2 tbsp.	51	2.6/.4	.6/1.5	1.6 *SOL	.14	na
EGG WHITES							
White	1 large	17	0/0	0/0	0	.23	55

* Assuming UNSALTED brands.
** Assuming these are homemade using non-iodized salt, or made with other LID-safe ingredients.

Food	Serving Size	Calories	Fat/Sat. Fat (gm)	Poly/Mono Unsaturated Fat (gm)	Fiber (gm)	Sugars (gm)	Sodium (mg)
FATS & OILS							
Beef tallow	1 tbsp.	115	13/6	.51/5.3	0	0	0
Lard	1 tbsp.	115	13/5	1.4/5.8	0	0	0
Shortening (Crisco)	1 tbsp.	110	12/3	na	0	0	na
Canola oil	1 tbsp.	122	13.6/1	4.1/8.2	0	0	na
Corn oil	1 tbsp.	120	14/2	7.4/3.7	0	0	na
Flaxseed oil**	1 tbsp.	120	13.6/1.3	9/2.7	0	0	na
Grapeseed oil	1 tbsp.	120	13.6/1.3	9.5/2.2	0	0	na
Olive oil	1 tbsp.	120	14/0	1.3/10	0	0	na
Peanut oil	1 tbsp.	122	13.6/2.5	4.3/6.2	0	0	na
Popcorn oil	1 tbsp.	120	14/2	4.3/6.2	0	0	na
Safflower oil, linoleic over 70%	1 tbsp.	120	13.6/.8	10/1.9	0	0	na
Sunflower oil	1 tbsp.	120	13.6/1.4	4.9/6.3	0	0	na
Vegetable oil	1 tbsp.	122	13.6/2	na	0	0	na
Wheat germ oil	1 tbsp.	120	13.6/2.5	8.4/2	0	0	na
FLOURS							
Barley flour	1 cup	511	2.3/.5	1.1/.3	4.4 *SOL	1.2	6
Blue corn flour	1 cup	520	6/0	na	12	na	na
Brown rice flour	1 cup	574	4.4/.9	1.6/1.6	7	120.8	13
Buckwheat flour	1 cup	402	3.7/.8	1.1/1.1	12	3.1	13
Carob flour	1 cup	229	.7/.09	.22/.2	41	50	36
Chickpea flour	1 cup	339	6/.6	2.7/1.4	10 *SOL	10	59
Corn flour, masa	1 cup	416	4/.6	2/1.1	11	.73	6

**Available in high-lignan formulations.

283

Food	Serving Size	Calories	Fat/Sat. Fat (gm)	Poly/Mono Unsaturated Fat (gm)	Fiber (gm)	Sugars (gm)	Sodium (mg)
FLOURS (continued)							
Corn flour, white, whole grain	1 cup	422	4.6/.6	2/1.2	11	.75	6
Corn flour, yellow, whole grain	1 cup	422	4.5/.6	2/1.2	16	.75	6
Graham flour	1 cup	360	20/0	na	16	na	na
Kamut flour	1 cup	440	0/0	na	16	na	na
Matzo meal	¼ cup	130	0/0	0/0	.01	1	0
Oat flour	1 cup	400	8/0	na	t	na	na
Oat bran flour	⅓ cup	76	2.2/.4	.9/.7	.67 *SOL	20	170
Peanut flour, defatted	1 cup	196	.3/.03	.08/.13	9.5	4.9	108
Peanut flour, low-fat	1 cup	257	13/2	4.1/6.5	9.5	18.76	1
Potato flour	1 cup	571	.5/.15	.24/.01	9	5.6	88
Rye flour, dark	1 cup	415	3.5/.4	1.5/.42	29	1.33	1
Rye flour, light	1 cup	374	1.4/.14	.58/16	15	1	2
Rye flour, medium	1 cup	361	1.8/.2	.79/.21	15	1	3
Spelt flour	1 cup	440	4/0	na	8	na	na
Sunflower seed flour	1 cup	209	1/.08	.56/.16	3	22.9	2
Triticale flour	1 cup	439	2.4/.4	na	19	na	na
White flour, all-purpose, enriched	1 cup	455	1/.2	.52/.1	3.4	.34	3
White flour, cake	1 cup	496	1/.2	.52/.1	2.4	.42	3
White flour, self-rising, enriched	1 cup	442	1/.2	.51/.1	3.4	.27	1588
White flour, tortilla	1 cup	450	12/4.5	1.7/5	na	74.5	751
White flour, unbleached	1 cup	455	1/.2	.51/.1	3.4	.34	3
White rice flour	1 cup	578	2/.6	.6/.7	4	.19	0
Whole wheat flour	1 cup	407	2/.4	.93/.28	15	.49	6

Food	Serving Size	Calories	Fat/Sat. Fat (gm)	Poly/Mono Unsaturated Fat (gm)	Fiber (gm)	Sugars (gm)	Sodium (mg)
GRAINS							
Barley, pearled, cooked	1 cup	193	.7/.15	.34/.09	6 *SOL	.44	5
Basmati rice, cooked	1 cup	230	4/0	na	0	na	na
Brown rice, instant (Minute Rice)	1 cup	240	2/0	na	0	na	na
Brown rice, long-grain, cooked	1 cup	216	2/.35	.63/.64	3.5	.68	2
Brown rice, medium-grain, cooked	1 cup	218	1.6/.3	.58/.58	3.5	45.8	10
Brown rice, short-grain, cooked	1 cup	na	na	na	na	na	na
Brown rice, Spanish, cooked	1 cup	260	2.5/.5	na	5	na	na
Bulgur, cooked	1 cup	151	.4/.07	.18/.06	8	.18	9
Corn bran	1 cup	170	.7/.1	.32/.18	65 *SOL	0	5
Couscous, cooked	1 cup	176	.25/.05	.1/.03	2	.16	8
Couscous pilaf mix, cooked	1 cup	196	0/0	na	0	na	na
Millet, cooked	1 cup	207	2/.3	na	2	na	na
Quinoa	1 cup	636	10/1	4/2.6	10	117	36
Rye	1 cup	566	4/.5	1.9/.5	25	1.76	10
Semolina	1 cup	601	1.75/.25	.71/2	6.5	121	2
Wheat bran	¼ cup	30	.6/.09	.3/.09	7 *SOL	.06	0
Wheat germ	2 tbsp.	50	.3/.2	.82/.2	2 *SOL	7.15	2
Wheat, hard red	1 cup	632	4/.6	1.2/3.8	23	.79	4
Wheat, hard white	1 cup	657	3/.5	1.4/3.9	na	.79	4
Wheat, soft red	1 cup	556	2.6/.5	2.9/3	21	124	3
Wheat, soft white	1 cup	571	3/.6	1.4/3.38	21	.69	3
Wheat, sprouted	1 cup	214	1.4/.2	.29/.3	1	45.9	17

Food	Serving Size	Calories	Fat/Sat. Fat (gm)	Poly/Mono Unsaturated Fat (gm)	Fiber (gm)	Sugars (gm)	Sodium (mg)
GRAINS (continued)							
White rice, instant, cooked	1 cup	162	.3/.1	.6/.16	1	.08	.07
White rice, long-grain, cooked w/ salt	1 cup	205	.44/.12	.12/.14	0	.08	604
White rice, medium-grain, cooked	1 cup	242	.4/.1	.1/.12	.6	58.9	0
White rice, short-grain, cooked	1 cup	242	.35/.09	.1/.1	na	33.2	0
White rice, Spanish or Mexican	1 cup	216	4/.6	na	3	na	na
Wild rice, cooked	1 cup	166	.6/.08	.35/.08	3	1.2	5
FRUITS							
Acerola cherries, raw	1 cup	31.4	.3/.1	na	1.1	na	na
Apple, raw (3 ¼" dia.), with skin	1 fruit	81	.36/.1	.1/.01	4 *SOL	22	2
Apple, raw (3 ¼" dia.), no skin	1 fruit	63	.34/t	.04/t	2 *SOL	12.9	0
Apple, dried	5 pieces	78	.1/t	.03/t	3 *SOL	18.3	28
Applesauce, w/o salt, sweetened	1 cup	194	.5/.1	.14/.02	3 *SOL	42	8
Applesauce, w/o salt, unsweetened	1 cup	105	.1/0	.03/t	3 *SOL	24.6	5
Apricot, raw	1 fruit	17	.14/0	.03/.06	.9	3.23	0
Apricots, canned, heavy syrup	1 cup	214	.21/0	.04/.08	4	51.3	10
Apricots, canned, juice pack	1 cup	117	.1/0	.02/.04	4	26.2	10
Apricots, canned, light syrup	1 cup	159	.1/0	.02/.05	4	37.7	10
Apricots, canned, water pack	1 cup	66	.4/0	.07/.17	4	11.6	17
Apricot, dried	10 halves	83	.16/0	.02/.17	3	18.6	14
Avocado, California	1 each	278	26.5/4.2	3.1/17	8.7	.52	14
Avocado, Florida	1 each	489	30/7.4	5/17	15	7.4	6
Banana (8" long)	1 fruit	109	.57/.2	.1/.04	3 *SOL	16.6	1
Banana chips, dried	10 chips	51	.9/.7	.06/.2	9 *SOL	3.5	1

Food	Serving Size	Calories	Fat/Sat. Fat (gm)	Poly/Mono Unsaturated Fat (gm)	Fiber (gm)	Sugars (gm)	Sodium (mg)
FRUITS (continued)							
Blackberries, raw	1 cup	75	.56/0	0/.07	7.6	7	1
Blueberries, raw	1 cup	81	.55/0	.2/.07	4	14.4	1
Blueberries, frozen, sweetened	1 cup	186	.3/0	.13/t	5	45	2
Blueberries, frozen, unsweetened	1 cup	79	1/0	.43/.14	4.2	13	2
Cherries, raw	10 cherries	49	0/0	0/0	1.5	13	5
Cherries, water pack	1 cup	114	.3/.1	.09/.08	2.7	25.4	2
Cranberries, raw	1 cup	46	.2/0	.05/.02	4	3.8	2
Currants, black	1 cup	123	t/0	t/t	5.4	17.2	2
Currants, red	1 cup	67	t/0	t/t	4.5	8.25	1
Dates, whole, without pits	5 dates	114	.19/t	t/t	3	79.76	4
Dates, chopped	1 cup	490	1/t	.03/.06	13	112.8	1
Figs, dried	2 figs	42	.16/.02	.06/.03	4.6	8	2
Figs, canned, light syrup	1 cup	174	.3/.1	.12/.05	4.5	46.7	3
Grapefruit, pink (3 ¾" diameter)	1 half	37	.12/0	.02/.01	1.3 *SOL	9	1
Grapefruit, white (3 ¾" dia.)	1 half	39	.12/0	.02/.01	1.3 *SOL	9	1
Grapefruit, canned sections, light syrup	1 cup	152	.25/0	.06/.03	1 *SOL	38	5
Grapefruit, canned sections, water pack	1 cup	88	.2/0	.06/.03	1 *SOL	21	5
Grapes, red	1 cup	114	.93/.3	.08/t	1.6	24.8	3
Grapes, white	1 cup	114	.93/.3	.08/t	1.6	24.8	3

Food	Serving Size	Calories	Fat/Sat. Fat (gm)	Poly/Mono Unsaturated Fat (gm)	Fiber (gm)	Sugars (gm)	Sodium (mg)
FRUITS (continued)							
Guava	1 medium	46	.5/.2	.2/.05	5	4.9	1
Kiwi fruit, raw	1 fruit	46	2.6/0	.2/.04	2.6	6.8	2
Lemon, raw, without peel	1 fruit	17	1.6/0	.05/t	1.6 * SOL	1.4	1
Mango, diced	1 cup	107	45.1/.1	.08/.17	3	24.4	3
Melon, Cantaloupe	1/8 melon	24	.19/0	.13/t	.55	12	25
Melon, Casaba	1 cup	44	.2/0	.07/t	1.4	9.7	na
Melon, Honeydew	1/8 melon	56	.2/0	.07/t	1	19	23
Nectarine (2 ½" diameter)	1 fruit	67	.63/.1	.15/.12	2 * SOL	10.7	0
Orange, medium	1 fruit	62	16/0	.03/.11	3 * SOL	12	0
Orange sections, canned, juice pack	1 cup	93	.3/0	na	3.4 * SOL	na	na
Orange sections, raw	1 cup	85	.22/0	.04/.11	4 * SOL	16.8	0
Papaya, diced	1 cup	55	.2/t	.04/.05	2.5	8.3	4
Papaya, whole	1 fruit	119	.43/t	.09/.1	5.5	17.9	9
Passion fruit	1 fruit	18	.1/0	na	2	na	na
Peaches, raw, medium	1 fruit	42	.25/.02	.08/.07	2	8.2	0
Peaches, canned, heavy syrup	1 cup	194	.26/t	.1/.09	3.4	45.4	10
Peaches, canned, juice pack	1 cup	109	.07/0	.04/.03	3	26	10
Peaches, canned, water pack	1 cup	59	.1/0	.07/.05	3	11.7	7
Peaches, dried	3 halves	93	.3/0	.15/.11	3	21.9	3
Peaches, frozen, sliced, sweetened	1 cup	235	.3/0	.16/.12	4.5	55	15
Peaches, frozen, sliced	1 cup	107	.2/0	na	5	na	na

Food	Serving Size	Calories	Fat/Sat. Fat (gm)	Poly/Mono Unsaturated Fat (gm)	Fiber (gm)	Sugars (gm)	Sodium (mg)
FRUITS (continued)							
Pears, raw, medium	1 fruit	98	.66/0	.05/.04	4 *SOL	16	2
Pears, canned, heavy syrup	1 cup	197	.35/0	.08/.07	4 *SOL	40.4	13
Pears, canned, juice pack	1 cup	124	.17/0	.04/.03	4 *SOL	24	10
Pears, canned, water pack	1 cup	71	.1/0	.02/.03	4 *SOL	15	5
Pears, dried	10 each	459	1/t	.3/.24	13 *SOL	104	11
Persimmons, medium	1 fruit	67	0/0	0/0	3.6	21	2
Pineapple, fresh chunks	1 cup	76	.67/0	.06/.02	2 *SOL	8.4	2
Pineapple, canned, heavy syrup	1 cup	195	.3/0	.1/.03	3 *SOL	42.9	3
Pineapple, canned, juice pack	1 cup	150	.2/0	.07/.02	2 *SOL	36	2
Pineapple, canned, light syrup	1 cup	131	.3/0	.1/.03	2 *SOL	31.9	3
Pineapple, canned, water pack	1 cup	79	.2/0	.08/.03	2 *SOL	18.4	2
Plantains, raw	1 fruit	218	.66/t	.1/.06	4 *SOL	26.8	7
Plantains, cooked	1 cup	176	.28/t	.05/.02	3.5 *SOL	21.6	8
Plums, raw, medium	1 fruit	36	.41/0	.03/.09	1	6.5	0
Plums, canned, heavy syrup	1 cup	230	.26/0	.05/.16	2.5	39.5	35
Plums, canned, juice pack	1 cup	146	.05/0	.01/.03	2.5	35.8	3
Plums, canned, light syrup	1 cup	159	.3/0	.06/.17	2.5	38.7	50
Plums, canned, water pack	1 cup	102	0/0	0/0	2.5	25	2
Pomegranate, raw	1 fruit	105	.5/.1	.1/.07	.9	25.5	5
Prunes, dried, pitted, uncooked	5 prunes	100	.22/0	.03/.02	3	16	1
Prunes, stewed	1 cup	265	.57/0	.15/.45	16	83	6
Raisins	1 packet	42	.06/t	t/t	na	8.3	2
Raspberries, raw	1 cup	60	.68/0	.38/.06	8	4.4	1

Food	Serving Size	Calories	Fat/Sat. Fat (gm)	Poly/Mono Unsaturated Fat (gm)	Fiber (gm)	Sugars (gm)	Sodium (mg)
FRUITS (continued)							
Raspberries, frozen, sweetened	1 cup	258	.4/0	.2/.04	11	54.4	3
Raspberries, frozen, unsweetened	1 cup	123	1.4/0	na	17	na	na
Rhubarb, canned, light syrup	1 cup	220	.2/.1	na	3.5	na	na
Rhubarb, cooked	1 cup	278	.5/.1	na	4	ns	na
Strawberries, raw	1 cup	50	.61/0	.26/.07	4	3.3	2
Strawberries, frozen, sweetened	1 cup	222	.33/0	.1/.03	5	10	4
Strawberries, frozen, unsweetened	1 cup	77	.2/0	.16/.05	5	61	8
Tangelo	1 cup	45	.1/0	na	2.3 *SOL	na	na
Tangerine, medium	1 fruit	37	.16/0	.05/.11	2 *SOL	8.9	2
Tangerine, mandarin	1 cup	154	.25/0	.05/.04	1.7 *SOL	39	15
Tangerine, canned in light syrup	1 cup	92	.1/0	.01/.11	1.7 *SOL	22	12
Watermelon	1 wedge	92	1/.1	.1/.1	1.4	17.7	3
GOOSE*							
Roasted, meat and skin	1 cup	427	31/10	3.5/14	0	0	98
Roasted, meat only	1 cup	340	18/6.5	2/.6	0	0	109
Pate	1 tbsp.	60	5.7/1.8	3.3/1.9	0	.61	91
LAMB*							
Chop	1 med. chop	345	27/12	na	0	0	na
Leg, roasted	3 oz.	199	12/6	.47/4.7	0	0	57
Rib, roasted	3 oz.	290	23/10	1.7/9.8	0	0	63
Shoulder, roasted	3 oz.	241	16.3/6.8	1.3/6.6	0	0	57
Sweetbreads	3 oz.	148	3.6/1.3	na	0	0	na

*Based on normal use of non-iodized salt.

Food	Serving Size	Calories	Fat/Sat. Fat (gm)	Poly/Mono Unsaturated Fat (gm)	Fiber (gm)	Sugars (gm)	Sodium (mg)
NUTS & SEEDS*							
Almonds, butter	1 tbsp.	101	9.5/.9	na	.6	na	na
Almonds, dry roasted, unsalted	22 nuts (1 oz.)	169	15/1	3.6/9.5	3.4	1.3	na
Almonds, oil roasted, unsalted	22 nuts (1 oz.)	172	16/1.2	3.8/9.7	3	1.3	na
Almonds, slivered	1 cup	624	55/4	13/34	13	5.2	na
Brazil nuts	6–8 nuts	186	19/5	5.8/6.9	1.5	.66	na
Cashews, butter	1 tbsp.	94	8/1.6	1.3/4.7	.32	.8	na
Cashews, dry roasted, unsalted	18 nuts (1oz.)	163	13/2.6	2.2/7.7	.85	1.4	na
Cashews, oil roasted, unsalted	18 nuts (1oz.)	164	14/3	2.4/7.3	1	1.4	na
Chestnuts	10 nuts	206	2/.3	.28/.6	4.3	49	3
Coconut, 2" x 2" x ½"	1 piece	159	15/13	.16/.6	4	2.8	9
Coconut, shredded, sweetened	1 oz.	135	9/8	na	1.2	na	na
Coconut, shredded, unsweetened	1 oz.	187	18/16	na	4.6	na	na
Flaxseed	1 tbsp.	59	4/.4	2.7/.8	3.4	.13	4
Hazelnuts	10 nuts	88	8.5/.6	1/6.4	1.4	.6	0
Macadamia nuts, dry roasted, unsalted	10–12 nuts (1 oz.)	203	22/4	.4/16.8	2.3	1.17	na
Mixed nuts, dry roasted, unsalted	1 oz.	168	15/2	3/8.9	2.5	1.32	na
Mixed nuts, oil roasted, unsalted	1 oz.	174	16/2.6	3.8/9	1.6	1.2	na
Peanuts, boiled	30 nuts (1oz.)	89	6/.9	1.9/3	2.5	.69	na
Peanuts, dry roasted, unsalted	1 oz.	166	14/2	4.4/6.8	2.3	1	na
Peanuts, honey roasted	1 oz.	153	14/2	na	2.3	1	na
Peanuts, oil roasted	1 oz.	163	14/2	4/7	2.6	4.9	na
Peanuts, Spanish, oil roasted	1 oz.	164	14/2	4.8/6.2	2.5	na	na

* Based on unsalted brands.

Food	Serving Size	Calories	Fat/Sat. Fat (gm)	Poly/Mono Unsaturated Fat (gm)	Fiber (gm)	Sugars (gm)	Sodium (mg)
NUTS & SEEDS* (continued)							
Peanut butter w/o salt	2 tbsp.	188.5	16/3	4.7/7.9	na	2.7	5
Pecans, dried, 1 oz.	20 halves	196	20/2	6/11.5	3	1.1	0
Pine nuts	10 nuts	6	1.2/.09	.6/.3	.1	.06	0
Pistachios, dry roasted	47 nuts (1oz.)	161	13/1.6	3.9/6.9	3	2.2	na
Pumpkin seeds, dried	1 oz.	146	12/2	5.4/3.7	1	.65	na
Sesame seeds, dry	1 tbsp.	47	4.4/.6	1.9/1.6	1	.04	2
Sunflower seeds, hulled, dry roasted	1 oz.	93	8/.8	9.3/2.7	1.4	.77	na
Sunflower seeds, hulled, oil roasted	1 oz.	105	10/1	9.7/2.3	1.2	.88	na
Tahini (sesame butter)	1 tbsp.	85.5	7/1	3.5/3	1.4	3	5
Walnuts, black, 1 oz.	14 halves	172	16/1	10/4	1.4	.31	1
Walnuts, English, 1 oz.	14 halves	185	18.5/1.7	13/2.5	2	.74	1
PASTA/NOODLES (cooked)							
Chinese noodles, chow mein	1 cup	237	14/2	7.8/3.5	2	.12	198
Corn-based pasta	1 cup	176	1/.14	.4/.3	7	39	0
Macaroni, elbow	1 cup	197	1/.3	.4/.1	2	.91	1
Macaroni, spinach	1 cup	191	.8/.1	na	5.4	na	na
Macaroni, vegetable	1 cup	171	.15/.02	.06/.02	6	1.1	8
Macaroni, elbows, whole wheat	1 cup	174	.75/.14	.3/.1	4	1.1	4
Pasta, fresh	1 cup	262	2/.3	.8/.2	na	49.8	12
Pasta, fresh, spinach	1 cup	260	2/.4	.4/.6	na	59	12

* Based on unsalted brands.

Food	Serving Size	Calories	Fat/Sat. Fat (gm)	Poly/Mono Unsaturated Fat (gm)	Fiber (gm)	Sugars (gm)	Sodium (mg)
PASTA/NOODLES (continued)							
Pasta, linguini	1 cup	197	.9/.1	na	2.4	na	na
Rice noodles	1 cup	192	.35/.04	.04/.05	2	43.8	33
Spaghetti, enriched	1 cup	197	1/.1	.4/.01	3	.9	140
Spaghetti, enriched, spinach	1 cup	182	.9/.12	.4/.1	na	36.6	20
Spaghetti, enriched, whole wheat	1 cup	174	.75/.14	.3/.1	6	1.1	4
PORK*							
Boneless	3 oz.	149	7.6/1.7	.7/2.9	0	0	1155
Canned, extra lean	3 oz.	142	7/2.4	.1/.6	0	0	356
Patty, grilled	1 patty	203	18/6.7	.4/6	0	0	58
Roasted, lean portion	3 oz.	206	14/5	1.5/6.7	0	0	1009
Center rib, broiled	3 oz.	224	13/4.8	1/5.8	0	0	53
Chop, lean, breaded or floured, broiled or baked	1 medium 5.5 oz.	207	8.4/3	na	0	0	na
Chop, lean, broiled or baked	1 med. 5.5 oz.	176	8/3	.7/3.8	0	0	50
Cutlet, lean broiled or baked	3 oz.	181	9/3	na	0	0	na
Ground patty	1 patty	297	21/8	2.6/10	0	0	85
Roast, lean, loin	3 oz.	122	5/1.7	.5/2.3	0	0	48
Roast, lean, shoulder	3 oz.	196	11.5/4	.9/5	0	0	68
Spareribs, lean	1 med. cut	161	7/3	na	0	0	na
Spareribs, lean	3 oz.	147	5/2	.46/2	0	0	47

*Assuming normal use of non-iodized salt.

Food	Serving Size	Calories	Fat/Sat. Fat (gm)	Poly/Mono Unsaturated Fat (gm)	Fiber (gm)	Sugars (gm)	Sodium (mg)
SALADS*							
Chef salad w/o dressing	1 cup	73	4/2	na	.6	na	na
Fruit salad w/citrus	1 cup	152	8/2	na	3 *SOL	21.6	50
Fruit salad w/o citrus	1 cup	184	8/2	na	4 *SOL	30.1	47
Mixed salad greens, raw, w/o dressing	1 cup	271	9/1	na	2	43	331
SNACKS, Chips – Unsalted**							
Apple chips (Weight Watchers)	1 pouch	50	1/0	na	0 *SOL	na	na
Banana chips	1 oz.	147	9.5/8	.18/.55	2	.02	na
Brown rice chips	1 oz.	130	5/0	na	0	na	na
Carrot chips	1 oz.	150	9/0	na	0 *SOL	na	na
Potato chips, baked	1 oz.	120	1/0	na	0	1.2	na
Potato chips, regular unsalted	1 oz.	100	4/0	na	9	.06	na
Tortilla chips, low-fat	10 chips	44	.5/0	.29/.17	.5	.09	na
Tortilla chips, nacho, baked	1 oz.	110	1/0	1/4.3	2	17.7	na
Tortilla chips, nacho, light	1 oz.	126	4/.8	.6/2.5	1.4	na	na
SNACKS, Grain Cakes – Unsalted							
Rice cakes, apple cinnamon	1	50	0/0	na	0	na	na
Rice cakes, brown rice, multigrain	1	35	.3/.05	.13/.1	3 *SOL	7.2	0
Rice cakes, brown rice, plain	1	35	.25/.05	.09/.09	.4	7.3	na
Rice cakes, brown rice, rye	1	35	.35/.05	.14/.12	.4	7.2	na
Rice cakes, brown rice, sesame	1	35	.35/.05	.1/.1	.5	7.3	na

*Assuming normal use of non-iodized salt.
** These are representative of many unsalted chips you can purchase; you can add your own non-iodized salt to many of these chips.

Food	Serving Size	Calories	Fat/Sat. Fat (gm)	Poly/Mono Unsaturated Fat (gm)	Fiber (gm)	Sugars (gm)	Sodium (mg)
SNACKS (continued)							
Rice cakes, corn (Quaker)	1	35	.2/0	.1/.1	.2	7.3	na
Popcorn*, air-popped	1 cup	31	.34/.05	.09/1.2	.66	0	24
Popcorn*, oil-popped	²/₃ cup	113	2.2/na	na	1.1	13.5	84
Trail mix, unsalted	½ cup	285	12/6	3.6/1.7	na	45.9	7
TOMATOES & TOMATO PRODUCTS							
Canned, chopped	½ cup	30	0/0	0	2	7.3	132
Canned, crushed	½ cup	29	.25/0	t/t	1.5	5.6	282
Canned, whole	½ cup	25	0/0	0	1	3	154
Fresh, boiled	½ cup	32	.5/.07	.24/.09	1.3	4.7	9
Paste, w/o salt	½ cup	107	.6/.13	.2/.08	5.9	13.6	128
Pizza sauce, homemade	¼ cup	34	7/.3	na	1.3	na	na
Puree	½ cup	50	.2/.02	na	2.5	na	na
Raw, cherry	1 cherry	4	.06/t	.02/t	.2	.45	1
Raw, green	1 medium	30	.25/.03	.1/.03	1.4	4.9	16
Raw, Italian	1 medium	13	.2/.02	.08/.03	.7	1.6	3
Raw, orange	1 medium	18	.2/.03	.08/.03	1	3.5	47
Raw, red	1 medium	26	.4/.05	.16/.06	1.4	3.2	6
Raw, yellow	1 medium	32	.6/.07	.2/.08	1.5	6.3	29
Sauce, canned, unsalted	1 cup	78	.3/.1	.04/.04	1.8	5.2	na
Ready-to-serve, unsalted gourmet brand or homemade	½ cup	45	.24/.03	.03/.8	1.8	5.2	na

* Assuming you add non-iodized salt to homemade batches.

Food	Serving Size	Calories	Fat/Sat. Fat (gm)	Poly/Mono Unsaturated Fat (gm)	Fiber (gm)	Sugars (gm)	Sodium (mg)
TURKEY*							
Roasted, breast (meat/skin)	100 gm	189	7.4/2	1.8/2.4	0	0	63
Roasted, dark meat	1 cup	262	10/3.4	3/2.3	0	0	111
Roasted, leg	1 leg	148	7/2	1.9/2	0	0	55
Roasted, light meat	1 cup	276	12/3	2.8/3.9	0	0	88
Giblets, simmered	1 cup	289	17/5.7	1.8/7.2	0	0	93
Patty, breaded, fried	1 patty	181	11.5/3	3/4.8	.3	0	512
Patty, cooked	1 patty (4 oz.)	193	11/3	na	0	0	na
VEAL*							
Blade, roasted	3 oz.	158	7/3	.54/2.7	0	0	85
Chop, broiled	1 med. chop	232	13/5.6	na	0	0	na
Cutlet, broiled	1 cutlet	136	4/1.6	na	0	0	na
Cutlet, breaded, fried	1 cutlet	194	8/2.6	na	.3	.57	455
Ground, broiled	3 oz.	146	6.4/2.5	.47/2.4	0	0	71
Liver, panfried	3 oz.	208	7.2/2.3	1.2/1.3	0	0	94
VEGETABLES & LEGUMES**							
Alfalfa sprouts, raw	1 cup	10	.2/.02	na	1	na	na
Artichoke, hearts, canned in water	²/₃ cup	44	0/0	0	6	na	na
Artichoke, hearts, cooked from frozen	3 oz.	30	0/0	0	4	.66	229
Artichoke, marinated	²/₃ cup	168	14/2	na	8	na	na
Artichoke, whole, globe, cooked	1 medium	60	.2/.04	.08/t	6.5	1.19	397
Arugula, raw, chopped	1 cup	5	.1/t	.03/t	.3	.2	3

*Based on normal use of non-iodized salt. **All canned foods based on unsalted brands.

Food	Serving Size	Calories	Fat/Sat. Fat (gm)	Poly/Mono Unsaturated Fat (gm)	Fiber (gm)	Sugars (gm)	Sodium (mg)
VEGETABLES & LEGUMES* (cont.)							
Asparagus, cooked, canned spears	6 each	21	.7/.2	.3/.02	2	1.14	na
Asparagus, cooked from fresh, cuts and tips	½ cup	22	.3/.06	1/t	1.5	2.5	3
Asparagus, cooked from fresh, spears	6 each	22	t/t	.08/t	2	1.8	2
Asparagus, from frozen, cuts and tips	½ cup	25	.4/.1	na	1.5	na	na
Asparagus from frozen, spears	6 each	25	t/t	t	2	3.6	7
Bamboo shoots, canned, drained slices	1 cup	15	.3/.06	.1/t	1	1.2	5
Beans ** – Cooked**							
Beans, adzuki, boiled	½ cup	147	.1/.04	na	8 *SOL	28.5	9
Beans, black beans, canned	½ cup	114	.4/.01	.1/.03	7.5 *SOL	20	na
Beans, black-eyed peas	½ cup	na	na	na	na	na	na
Beans, chickpeas (garbanzo), canned	½ cup	135	2/.2	.6/.3	7 *SOL	27	na
Beans, fava, canned	½ cup	135	.2/.04	.11/.6	5 *SOL	15.9	580
Beans, great northern, canned	½ cup	91	.5/.1	.21/.2	7 *SOL	27.5	na
Beans, kidney, boiled	½ cup	149	.4/.06	.2/.29	7 *SOL	2.3	379
Beans, kidney, canned	½ cup	113	.4/.05	.24/.03	4.5 *SOL	.28	na
Beans, lima, boiled	½ cup	104	.25/.05	.13/.02	5 *SOL	1.39	215
Beans, lima, canned	½ cup	105	.4/.08	na	5 *SOL	na	na
Beans, lima, cooked from frozen	½ cup	88	.3/.06	.14/t	5 *SOL	1.14	246

*Based on normal use of non-iodized salt. **All canned foods based on unsalted brands.

Food	Serving Size	Calories	Fat/Sat. Fat (gm)	Poly/Mono Unsaturated Fat (gm)	Fiber (gm)	Sugars (gm)	Sodium (mg)
VEGETABLES & LEGUMES* (cont.)							
Beans, mung, boiled	½ cup	85	.3/.1	.13/.05	8 *SOL	2	240
Beans, navy, boiled	½ cup	106	.5/.1	.3/.09	6 *SOL	.34	216
Beans, navy, canned	½ cup	129	.5/.1	.24/.05	7 *SOL	.37	na
Beans, pinto, boiled	½ cup	148	.4/.09	.16/.11	7 *SOL	22.4	203
Beans, pinto, canned	½ cup	117	1/.2	.35/.2	5.5 *SOL	.26	na
Beans, white, boiled	½ cup	18	.3/.08	.25/.05	5.5 *SOL	23	213
Beans, white, canned	½ cup	125	.4/.1	.16/.03	7 *SOL	28.7	na
Beans – Fresh							
Snap, green string, French style, canned	½ cup	103	.1/.03	.12/t	2 *SOL	3.9	na
Snap, green string, French style, from fresh	½ cup	18	.1/.04	.03/t	2 *SOL	.77	3
Snap, green string, French style, from frozen	½ cup	22	.1/.03	.06/t	2 *SOL	.83	6
Snap, yellow, canned	½ cup	18	.1/.03	.03/t	2 *SOL	3.06	na
Snap, yellow, from fresh	½ cup	18	.1/.04	.03/t	2 *SOL	3.9	3
Snap, yellow, from frozen	½ cup	22	.1/.02	.05/t	2 *SOL	4.35	165
Bean sprouts (mung), raw	1 cup	31	.2/.05	na	2	na	na
Bean sprouts (mung), canned	1 cup	15	.08/.02	na	1	na	na

*All canned foods based on unsalted brands.

Food	Serving Size	Calories	Fat/Sat. Fat (gm)	Poly/Mono Unsaturated Fat (gm)	Fiber (gm)	Sugars (gm)	Sodium (mg)
VEGETABLES & LEGUMES* (cont.)							
Beets, raw	2 each	70	.3/.04	.1/.05	5	11	128
Beets, canned, sliced	½ cup	26	.1/.02	.04/.02	1.5	4.7	165
Beets, cooked from fresh, sliced	½ cup	37	.15/.02	.05/.03	2	6.8	65
Beets, pickled slices	½ cup	74	.09/.01	.03/.02	3	18.5	300
Beets, whole, canned	1 cup	51	.3/.03	.06/.03	3	16	352
Beets, whole, cooked from fresh	2 each	44	.2/.03	.06/.03	2	7.9	77
Beet greens, cooked	½ cup	20	.14/.02	.05/.03	2	3.9	343
Breadfruit, cooked	½ cup	145	.3/.1	na	7	na	na
Broccoli, raw, chopped	1 cup	25	.3/.05	.03/.01	2.6	1.5	29
Broccoli, raw, spears	2 each	18	.05/t	.0/2	2	1	20
Broccoli, cooked from fresh, chopped	½ cup	22	.3/.04	.13/t	2	1	204
Broccoli, cooked from fresh, spears	2 each	21	.3/.04	.12/.02	2	1	194
Broccoli, cooked from frozen, chopped	½ cup	25	.1/.01	.05/t	2	1.3	239
Broccoli, cooked from frozen, spears	½ cup	26	.1/.01	.05/t	3	1.3	239
Broccoflower, raw	1 cup	20	.2/0	.12/.02	2	3.7	19
Broccoflower, cooked	½ cup	14	.1/0	na	1.5	na	na
Brussel sprouts, cooked from fresh	½ cup	32	.4/.08	.2/.03	2	6.7	200
Brussel sprouts, cooked from frozen	½ cup	33	.3/.02	.02/.03	3	6.4	201

*Assuming all are cooked with average quantities of non-iodized salt; all canned foods based on unsalted brands.

Food	Serving Size	Calories	Fat/Sat. Fat (gm)	Poly/Mono Unsaturated Fat (gm)	Fiber (gm)	Sugars (gm)	Sodium (mg)
VEGETABLES & LEGUMES* (cont.)							
Cabbage, common varieties, raw, shredded, or chopped	1 cup	22	.2/.03	.04/t	2	2.5	13
Cabbage, common varieties, cooked, drained	½ cup	17	.3/.04	.07/.01	2	3.5	183
Cabbage, bok choy, raw, shredded	1 cup	9	.1/.01	.07/.01	.7	.83	46
Cabbage, bok choy, cooked	½ cup	10	.1/.01	.06/.01	1.5	.7	230
Cabbage, red, raw chopped	1 cup	19	.2/.02	.11/.05	1.4	3.5	24
Cabbage, red, cooked, drained	½ cup	16	.15/.02	.07/.01	1.5	3.5	183
Cabbage, savoy, raw, chopped	1 cup	19	.07/t	.03/t	2	1.6	20
Cabbage, savoy, cooked, drained	½ cup	17	.05/t	.03/t	2	3.9	189
Capers	1 tbsp.	2	.07/.02	.03/t	.3	.04	255
Carrots, fresh, grated	1 cup	47	.2/.03	.13/.01	3 *SOL	5	76
Carrots, fresh, whole	1 medium	26	.1/.02	.08/.01	2 *SOL	3.3	50
Carrots, sliced, canned	½ cup	28	.2/.03	.08/t	2 *SOL	3	na
Carrots, sliced, cooked from fresh, drained	½ cup	35	.1/.02	.07/t	2.5 *SOL	2.7	236
Carrots, sliced, cooked from frozen, drained	½ cup	26	.08/.01	.23/.03	2.5 *SOL	2.9	215
Carrots, baby, raw	4 medium	15	.2/.04	.03/t	7 *SOL	1.9	31
Carrots, baby, cooked from frozen	⅔ cup	35	0/0	na	2 *SOL	na	na
Cauliflower, raw	1 cup	25	.2/.03	.1/.01	2.5	2.4	30
Cauliflower, cooked from fresh, drained	½ cup	14	.3/.04	.12/.02	2	.87	150
Cauliflower, cooked from frozen, drained	½ cup	17	.2/.03	.09/.01	2.5	.94	229

*Assuming all are cooked with average quantities of non-iodized salt; all canned foods based on unsalted brands.

Food	Serving Size	Calories	Fat/Sat. Fat (gm)	Poly/Mono Unsaturated Fat (gm)	Fiber (gm)	Sugars (gm)	Sodium (mg)
VEGETABLES & LEGUMES* (cont.)							
Celery, raw	1 med. stalk	6	.06/.02	.03/.01	.7	.73	32
Celery, cooked from fresh	½ cup	13	.1/.03	.03/t	1	.11	245
Celeriac root, cooked	½ cup	21	.15/0	na	.5	4.6	230
Chard, Swiss, raw	1 cup	7	.6/.01	.02/.01	.6	.4	77
Chard, Swiss, cooked from fresh	½ cup	17	.07/0	na	2	.96	363
Chayote, raw	1 chayote	39	.3/.06	.11/.02	3.5	3.8	4
Chayote, cooked	½ cup	19	.3/.07	na	2	4	190
Collards, cooked from fresh	½ cup	25	.3/.04	.16/.02	2.5	4.7	239
Collards, cooked from frozen	½ cup	30	.35/.05	na	2.5	.48	243
Corn (white), canned	½ cup	66	.8/.1	.25/.15	1.5	20.8	na
Corn (white), cob cooked from fresh	1 ear	96	1/.2	.54/.3	2	3.6	225
Corn (white), cob cooked from frozen	1 ear	68	.4/.1	.22/.1	2	14	151
Corn (white), kernals, cooked from frozen	½ cup	66	.35/.05	.2/.2	2	16	201
Corn (yellow), canned	½ cup	83	.5/.08	.3/.18	2	3.6	193
Corn (yellow), cob cooked from fresh	1 ear	83	1/.15	.5/.3	2	2.8	225
Corn (yellow), cob cooked from frozen	1 ear	68	.4/.1	.22/.1	2	2.3	151
Corn (yellow), kernels, cooked from frozen	½ cup	82	.6/.09	.25/.16	2	4.1	365

*Assuming all are cooked with average quantities of non-iodized salt; all canned foods based on unsalted brands.

Chapter 10: Nutritional Analysis Chart

Food	Serving Size	Calories	Fat/Sat. Fat (gm)	Poly/Mono Unsaturated Fat (gm)	Fiber (gm)	Sugars (gm)	Sodium (mg)
VEGETABLES & LEGUMES* (cont.)							
Cucumber slices w/peel	1 cup	14	.1/.02	.03/.0	.8	.87	1
Cucumber slices w/o peel	1 cup	14	.2/.05	t/t	1	1.6	2
Dandelion greens, raw	1 cup	25	.4/.09	.17/t	2	2.1	42
Dandelion greens, cooked	½ cup	17	.3/.07	na	1.5	1.4	147
Eggplant, boiled	1 cup	28	.2/.04	.04/.02	2.5	na	237
Eggplant, cubed, raw	1 cup	21	.15/.03	.06/.01	2	na	2
Endive, fresh, chopped	1 cup	8.5	.1/.02	.02/t	1.5	na	6
Grape leaves, raw	1 cup	13	.3/.05	.15/.01	1.5	na	1
Jicama, raw	1 cup	49	.1/.03	.06/t	6	na	5
Kale, raw, chopped	1 cup	34	.5/.06	.23/t	1	na	29
Kale, cooked from fresh	½ cup	19.5	.3/.4	.25/.04	1	na	337
Kale, cooked from frozen	½ cup	19.5	.3/t	.3/.05	1	na	326
Kohlrabi, raw	1 cup	36	.1/.01	.06/t	5	na	27
Kohlrabi, cooked	½ cup	24	.09/t	.04/t	1	na	212
Leeks, raw (bulb, lower leaves)	1 leek	54	.3/.04	.15/t	1.6	na	18
Leeks, cooked (bulb, lower leaves)	1 leek	38	.25/.03	.14/t	1	na	305
Lentils, cooked from dry	½ cup	115	.3/.05	.17/.06	8 *SOL	na	236
Lentils, sprouted	1 cup	82	.4/.04	.17/.06	3 *SOL	na	8
Lettuce, raw, chopped, Boston/butterhead	1 cup	7	.1/.01	.06/t	.6	na	3
Lettuce, raw, chopped, escarole	1 cup	8	t/t	t/t	1	na	na
Lettuce, raw, chopped, iceberg	1 cup	7	.1/.01	.05/t	.8	na	7
Lettuce, raw, chopped, looseleaf	1 cup	10	.2/.02	.03/t	1	na	10

*Assuming all are cooked with average quantities of non-iodized salt.

Food	Serving Size	Calories	Fat/Sat. Fat (gm)	Poly/Mono Unsaturated Fat (gm)	Fiber (gm)	Sugars (gm)	Sodium (mg)
VEGETABLES & LEGUMES* (cont.)							
Lettuce, raw, chopped, radicchio	1 cup	9	.1/.02	na	.4	na	na
Lettuce, raw, chopped, romaine	1 cup	8	t/t	t/t	1	na	4
Mushrooms, raw, common types, sliced	1 cup	18	.2/.03	.09/t	.9	1.3	220
Mushrooms, canned, common types	½ cup, pieces	19	.2/.03	.09/t	2	1.7	na
Mushrooms, cooked from raw	½ cup, pieces	21	.4/.05	.14/t	2	1.7	186
Mushrooms, oyster, raw	1 large	55	.8/0	na	4	na	na
Mushrooms, portobello, raw	3.5 oz.	26	.2/.03	.08/t	1.5	1.8	6
Mushrooms, shiitake, cooked	½ cup, pieces	40	.2/.04	.02/.05	1.5	10.3	174
Mushrooms, shiitake, dried	4 'shrooms	44	.15/.04	.02/.05	2	3.4	2
Okra, raw	1 cup	33	.1/.03	.03/.02	3	1.2	8
Okra, cooked from fresh, sliced	½ cup	26	.1/.04	.03/.04	2	3.6	193
Okra, cooked from frozen, sliced	½ cup	34	.1/t	t/t	3	2.6	220
Onions, raw	1 medium	42	.2/.03	.1/.04	2	6.8	5
Onions, raw, chopped	½ cup	31	.1/.02	.07/.02	1.5	4.7	3
Onions, cooked	½ cup	46	.2/.03	t/t	1.5	.34	18
Onions, green, spring, chopped (bulb/top)	½ cup	16	t/t	t/t	1	1.2	8
Onions, flakes, dehydrated	1 tbsp.	17	t/t	t/t	.5	1.8	1

*Assuming all are cooked with average quantities of non-iodized salt; all canned foods based on unsalted brands.

Food	Serving Size	Calories	Fat/Sat. Fat (gm)	Poly/Mono Unsaturated Fat (gm)	Fiber (gm)	Sugars (gm)	Sodium (mg)
VEGETABLES & LEGUMES* (cont.)							
Parsley, raw, chopped	½ cup	11	.2/.03	.04/.09	1	.26	17
Parsley, raw, sprigs	5 sprigs	2	t/t	t/t	.1	0	0
Parsnips, cooked, sliced	½ cup	63	.2/.04	.04/t	3	15.2	192
Peas, green, canned	½ cup	59	.3/.05	.14/.03	3.5 *SOL	3.5	214
Peas, green, cooked from fresh	½ cup	62	.2/.04	.08/.01	4 *SOL	4.7	191
Peas, green cooked from frozen	½ cup	62	.2/.04	.1/.02	4 *SOL	11.4	258
Peas, pod peas, edible, cooked	½ cup	33	t/t	t/t	2 *SOL	na	na
Peas, Split peas, cooked from dry	½ cup	115	.4/.05	.16/.08	8 *SOL	2.8	233
Peppers, banana, raw	1 medium	12	.2/.02	.11/.01	1.5	.9	6
Peppers, chili, green, canned	½ cup	14	.07/t	.1/.01	1	3.2	276
Peppers, chili, green, raw	1 medium	18	.09/t	t/t	.7	2.3	3
Peppers, chili, red, canned	½ cup	14	.07/t	t/t	1	1.2	428
Peppers, chili, red, raw	1 medium	18	.09/t	.1/t	.7	2.4	4
Peppers, jalapeno, sliced canned	½ cup	14	.5/.05	.04/t	3	.48	0
Peppers, jalapeno, raw	1 medium	18	.1/0	.35/.04	.7	1.5	1136
Peppers, sweet, green, raw	1 medium	32	.2/.03	.07/.01	2	2.9	4
Peppers, sweet, green, cooked, chopped	½ cup	19	.1/.02	.1/.01	.8	6.2	219
Peppers, sweet, red, raw	1 medium	32	.2/.03	.19/t	.2	5	2
Peppers, sweet, red, cooked, chopped	½ cup	19	.1/.02	.09/t	.8	6.2	219
Peppers, sweet, red, marinated	1 oz.	10	0/0	0	t	2.7	958

*Assuming all are cooked with average quantities of non-iodized salt; all canned foods based on unsalted brands.

Food	Serving Size	Calories	Fat/Sat. Fat (gm)	Poly/Mono Unsaturated Fat (gm)	Fiber (gm)	Sugars (gm)	Sodium (mg)
VEGETABLES & LEGUMES* (cont.)							
Peppers, sweet, yellow, raw	1 large	50	.4/.06	na	2	11.7	4
Peppers, sweet, yellow, strips	10 strips	14	.1/.02	na	.5	3.3	1
Potatoes, baked w/skin	1 medium	220	t/t	t/t	5	36.6	8
Potatoes, baked w/o skin	1 medium	145	t/t	t/t	2	33.6	8
Potatoes, boiled w/o skin	1 medium	116	t/t	t/t	2	33.4	402
Potatoes, microwaved w/skin	1 medium	212	t/t	t/t	5	15.6	16
Pumpkin, mashed, canned	½ cup	41	.03/.01	.02/.04	3.5	9.9	na
Pumpkin, mashed, cooked from fresh	½ cup	25	.08/.04	t/.01	1.5	1.2	290
Radishes, raw	½ cup	12	.3/.02	.03/.01	1	1.2	23
Rutabaga, cooked, mashed	½ cup	47	.3/.04	.11/.03	2	7.2	305
Shallots, raw	1 tbsp.	7	.01/t	t/t	t	1.7	1
Spinach, raw	1 cup	7	.1/.02	.05/t	1	.13	24
Spinach, canned	½ cup	25	.5/.08	.18/.01	2.5	3.4	na
Spinach, cooked from fresh	½ cup	20	.25/.03	.1/t	2	3.4	275
Spinach, cooked from frozen	½ cup	27	.2/.03	.2/0	3	4.9	306
Squash, summer, yellow, raw	1 cup	23	.2/.05	.1/.02	2	2.5	2
Squash, summer, yellow, cooked	½ cup	14	.07/.1	.12/.02	1.5	2.3	213
Squash, summer, zucchini, raw	1 cup	17	.2/.04	.02/t	1.5	1.5	215
Squash, summer, zucchini, cooked	½ cup	14	.04/t	.09/.02	1.2	2.1	12

*Assuming all are cooked with average quantities of non-iodized salt; all canned foods based on unsalted brands.

Food	Serving Size	Calories	Fat/Sat. Fat (gm)	Poly/Mono Unsaturated Fat (gm)	Fiber (gm)	Sugars (gm)	Sodium (mg)
VEGETABLES & LEGUMES* (cont.)							
Squash, winter, acorn, mashed, w/o salt	½ cup	41	.1/.03	.04/t	3	10.8	4
Squash, winter, butternut, mashed w/o salt	½ cup	47	.08/.01	.04/t	3	10.7	4
Squash, winter, hubbard, mashed w/o salt	½ cup	35	.4/.1	.37/.07	3.5	15.2	12
Squash, winter, spaghetti, baked w/o salt	1 cup	42	.4/.1	.19/.03	2	10	394
Sweet potato, baked in skin	1 medium	117	.1/.03	.1/t	3.5	9.6	41
Sweet potato, canned, pieces	1 cup	344	1/.02	.2/.02	6	10	na
Sweet potato, mashed	1 cup	182	.4/.09	.26/0	3.6	18.8	89
Taro shoots, cooked slices	½ cup	10	.05/.01	.02/t	na	2.2	167
Tomatillos, raw, each	1 medium	11	.4/.05	.14/.05	.7	1.3	0
Tomatillos, raw, chopped	1 cup	42	1/.2	.5/.2	2.5	5	1
Turnips, cooked, mashed	1 cup	48	.2/.02	.1/.01	5	11.3	658
Turnip greens, cooked from fresh	½ cup	25	.3/.08	.07/.01	3	.38	191
Turnip greens, cooked from frozen	½ cup	25	.4/.08	.06/t	3	.87	205
Water chestnuts, canned, slices	½ cup	35	.04/.01	na	2	na	na
Water chestnuts, canned, whole	4 each	14	.02/t	na	.7	na	na
Watercress, raw, chopped	1 cup	4	.03/t	.01/t	.5	.07	14
VEGETABLES MIXED							
Broccoli, corn, and red pepper	½ cup	60	1/0	na	3	na	na
Brussels sprouts, cauliflower, and carrots	½ cup	40	0/0	na	4	na	na

*Assuming all are cooked with average quantities of non-iodized salt; all canned foods based on unsalted brands.

Food	Serving Size	Calories	Fat/Sat. Fat (gm)	Poly/Mono Unsaturated Fat (gm)	Fiber (gm)	Sugars (gm)	Sodium (mg)
VEGETABLES MIXED * (cont.)							
Cauliflower, zucchini, carrots, red pepper	½ cup	30	0/0	na	2	na	na
Corn w/ peppers (Mexican corn)	½ cup	89	1/.2	na	2	na	na
Green beans and almonds	½ cup	97	7/.7	na	2	na	na
Green beans and onions	½ cup	23	.1/0	na	2	na	na
Green beans and potatoes	½ cup	41	.1/0	na	2	na	na
Green beans and tomatoes	½ cup	25	.2/0	na	2	na	na
Mixed vegetables, canned	½ cup	43	.2/0	.1/.01	3	7.5	121
Mixed vegetables, from frozen	½ cup	54	.1/0	t/t	4	11.9	247
Mixed vegetables, from frozen California blend (Freshlike)	½ cup	30	0/0	na	t	na	na
Mixed vegetables, from frozen Italian blend (Freshlike)	½ cup	30	0/0	na	t	na	na
Oriental-style mixed vegetables	½ cup	24	.1/0	na	2	na	na
Peas and carrots, canned	½ cup	50	0/0	0	t	10.8	na
Peas and carrots, from frozen	½ cup	38	.3/.06	.16/.03	t	8.1	243
Peas and corn	½ cup	78	.6/.1	na	3	na	na
Peas and mushrooms	½ cup	54	.2/0	na	4	na	na
Peas and onions	½ cup	41	.2/0	na	2	na	na
Peas and potatoes	½ cup	67	.1/0	na	3	na	na
Ratatouille	½ cup	76	6/.8	na	2	na	na
Succotash	½ cup	89	.9/.2	.4/.15	4 *SOL	23.4	243

*Assuming all are cooked with average quantities of non-iodized salt; all canned foods based on unsalted brands.

Food	Serving Size	Calories	Fat/Sat. Fat (gm)	Poly/Mono Unsaturated Fat (gm)	Fiber (gm)	Sugars (gm)	Sodium (mg)
VEGETABLES MIXED* (cont.)							
Summer squash and onions	½ cup	27	.2/0	na	1	na	na
Vegetable and pasta combination	½ cup	90	4/1	na	.6	na	na
Vegetables, stew type	½ cup	39	.1/0	na	2	na	na
Vegetable, stir-fry	½ cup	34	.05/0	na	1	na	na
Zucchini w/tomato sauce	½ cup	20	.1/0	na	2	na	na

*Assuming all are cooked with average quantities of non-iodized salt; all canned foods based on unsalted brands.

Sources Used to Create This Chart:

1. U.S. Department of Agriculture Nutrient Data Laboratory. *USDA National Nutrient Database for Standard Reference,* Release 17. Beltsville, Maryland.

2. U.S. Food and Drug Administration Center for Food Safety and Applied Nutrition. 2003. *Guidance on How to Understand and Use the Nutrition Facts Panel on Food Labels,* (June 2000; Updated July 2003). Online: www.cfsan.fda.gov/~dms/foodlab.html

RECIPE INDEX

Recipe Index

Beef broth, 128
Beet soup, chilled, 82
Black bean and corn casserole, 109
Black bean soup, 122
Blueberry apple crisp, 221
Blueberry apple pie, 216
Blueberry orange muffins, 66
Blueberry pancakes, 61
Brisket, 167, 169, 176
Broccoli pancakes, 96
Broth, 128, 134
Bruschetta, tomato and basil, 259

C

Cabbage rolls, 110
Cabbage soup with meatballs, 79
Cajun seasoning, 243
Carrot cake, 205
Carrot muffins, 72
Carrots-for-breakfast pancakes, 62
Cashew milk, 52
Chicken dinner, quick, 153
Chicken with fettuccine, 193
Chicken fillets, breaded, 148
Chicken fingers, 151
Chicken kabobs, grilled, 154, 160
Chicken, lima bean and barley soup, 124
Chicken livers, 164
Chicken primavera, 187
Chicken and rice casserole, 150
Chicken soup, 83, 133
Chicken spaghetti soup, 80

Made in the USA
Las Vegas, NV
12 February 2024

85708674R00177